"Dr. Sheppard and Dr. Thieneman are experts in both the theory AND practice of group therapy. This book represents a rare find: A bridge between important-but-dense academic research articles and actual real-world practice, with rich case examples and examples of therapeutic dialogue that would benefit any practitioner, from neophyte to expert."

DeDe Wohlfarth, *PsyD, Full Professor of Psychology, Spalding University, Licensed Clinical Psychologist, IN and KY*

"These two gifted child group therapists have added immeasurably to our field with this book. Their contribution, which draws on their many years of child group work, weaves together technique and theory and is a valuable resource to experienced and beginning clinicians alike."

Seth Aronson, *PsyD, CGP, AGPA-F, William Alanson White Institute, USA*

"A much needed guide – theoretically grounded, practically oriented, and easy to read – to working with children in therapy groups. A heartfelt thankyou to the authors!"

Thomas Hurster, *MSS, LCSW, AGPA-F, Bryn Mawr College Graduate School of Social Work and Social Research, USA*

Group Psychotherapy with Children

This book guides the reader through the process of creating evidence-based therapy groups for children.

Introducing an interpersonal theoretical framework that maximizes the interactional and experiential learning and growth components of groups with children, this curriculum offers the child group therapist a theoretical foundation that gives structure to existing techniques and an approach that is multiculturally sensitive and grounded in brain science. A deeper understanding of the mechanisms of change that operate in children's groups is central to the theme, including an emphasis on play and "learning by doing" through real-life clinical examples that permit readers of all levels to achieve a better understanding of how child groups function.

Readers of this book will come away with a deeper understanding of the "power cell" of group therapy: Working interpersonally in the here and now, specifically with children.

Tony L. Sheppard, PsyD, CGP, ABPP, AGPA-F, is a psychologist in private practice and has been involved in group work with children and adolescents for over 20 years.

Zachary J. Thieneman, PsyD, CGP, is a psychologist in private practice and has worked with children and adolescents for over 15 years.

AGPA Group Therapy Training and Practice Series

Series Editors: Les Greene and Rebecca MacNair-Semands

The American Group Psychotherapy Association (AGPA) is the foremost professional association dedicated to the field of group psychotherapy, operating through a tri-partite structure: AGPA, a professional and educational organization; the Group Foundation for Advancing Mental Health, its philanthropic arm; and the International Board for Certification of Group Psychotherapists, a standard setting and certifying body. This multidisciplinary association has approximately 3,000 members, including psychiatrists, psychologists, social workers, nurses, clinical mental health counselors, marriage and family therapists, pastoral counselors, occupational therapists and creative arts therapists, many of whom have been recognized as specialists through the Certified Group Psychotherapist credential. The association has 26 local and regional societies located across the country. Its members are experienced mental health professionals who lead psychotherapy groups and various non-clinical groups. Many are organizational specialists who work with businesses, not-for-profit organizations, communities and other "natural" groups to help them improve their functioning.

The goal of the AGPA Group Therapy Training and Practice Series is to produce the highest quality publications to aid the practitioner and student in updating and improving his/her knowledge, professional competence and skills with current and new developments in methods, practice, theory, and research in the group psychotherapy field. Books in this series are the only curriculum guide and resource for a variety of courses credentialed by the International Board for Certification of Group Psychotherapists. While this is the series' original and primary purpose, the texts are also useful in a variety of other settings including as a resource for students and clinicians interested in learning more about group psychotherapy, as a text in academic courses, or as part of a training curriculum in a practicum or internship training experience.

Books in this Series:

Group Psychotherapy Assessment and Practice:
A Measurement-Based Care Approach,
Martyn Whittingham and Rebecca MacNair-Semands

Group Psychotherapy with Children:
Core Principles for Effective Practice,
Tony L. Sheppard and Zachary J. Thieneman

For more information about this series, please visit https://www.routledge.com/AGPA-Group-Therapy-Training-and-Practice-Series/book-series/AGPA.

Group Psychotherapy with Children

Core Principles for Effective Practice

**Tony L. Sheppard and
Zachary J. Thieneman**

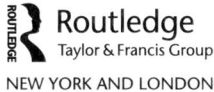

Routledge
Taylor & Francis Group

NEW YORK AND LONDON

Cover image designed by © Getty Image

First published 2024
by Routledge
605 Third Avenue, New York, NY 10158

and by Routledge
4 Park Square, Milton Park, Abingdon, Oxon, OX14 4RN

Routledge is an imprint of the Taylor & Francis Group, an informa business

© 2024 Tony L. Sheppard and Zachary J. Thieneman

Library of Congress Cataloging-in-Publication Data
Names: Sheppard, Tony L., author. | Thieneman, Zachary J., author.
Title: Group psychotherapy with children: core principles for effective
practice / by Tony L. Sheppard and Zachary J. Thieneman.
Description: New York, NY: Routledge, 2024. | Series: AGPA group therapy
training and practice series | Includes bibliographical references and index. |
Identifiers: LCCN 2023008361 (print) | LCCN 2023008362 (ebook) |
ISBN 9781032039190 (hardback) | ISBN 9781032039183 (paperback) |
ISBN 9781003189701 (ebook)
Subjects: LCSH: Group psychotherapy for children. | Group psychotherapy
for youth.
Classification: LCC RJ505.G7 S527 2024 (print) | LCC RJ505.G7 (ebook) |
DDC 618.92/89152–dc23/eng/20230601
LC record available at https://lccn.loc.gov/2023008361
LC ebook record available at https://lccn.loc.gov/2023008362

ISBN: 978-1-032-03919-0 (hbk)
ISBN: 978-1-032-03918-3 (pbk)
ISBN: 978-1-003-18970-1 (ebk)

DOI: 10.4324/9781003189701

Typeset in Baskerville
by codeMantra

Contents

Acknowledgments

As the authors of this work, we would like to thank the American Group Psychotherapy Association and its staff for their guidance in producing this book. The American Group Psychotherapy Association's Science to Service Task Force was invaluable in helping us get this project to the page. We particularly want to thank Task Force Co-Chairs, Rebecca MacNair-Semands, Les Greene, and Cheri Marmarosh. Reviews by Tom Hurster, Seth Aronson and Dede Wohlfarth vastly enhanced the content that ended up on these pages. Further, we must thank and acknowledge our many group members, graduate students (especially Beth Curran for her work on our appendices), teachers, mentors, and friends from across the years. Each of these people contributed to our knowledge about group work with children. Finally, we must thank our families for permitting us the time away from them to write and edit for the duration of this project. Our partners, Rachel (TLS) and Kate (ZJT), and children Lydia and Matthew (TLS) and Maddox (ZJT) gave us the inspiration to bring this project to fruition. Without their continued support, this project would remain incomplete.

It is our hope that the readers of this curriculum find passion and excitement for group psychotherapy with children. This curriculum is born out of our own enthusiasm for child groups and the magical properties they hold. We truly hope that it inspires your work and helps you to engage in becoming the best child group therapist you can be.

1 Foundations of Group Psychotherapy with Children

Tony L. Sheppard

Introduction

Group psychotherapy represents an indispensable modality in the treatment of children. Myriad problems faced by children are amenable to treatment in groups. In fact, group treatment is a preferred modality for many presenting problems and in many settings. Therapy groups for children can be found in a variety of settings including outpatient mental health clinics, private practices, inpatient centers, residential facilities and schools. Schaefer (1999) provides a compelling rationale for the use of group therapy for children as he states, "Of all the psychotherapy modalities, group therapy, in particular, complements the normal developmental tasks that further children's capacities for social interaction and intimacy" (p. vii). We are, after all, social creatures, and group therapy is our most social of therapeutic interventions. Kratochwill and Stoiber (1998) cite a number of societal changes that make group therapy a primary component of a successful and efficient mental healthcare delivery system in the treatment of children. Among these societal changes are the increasing number of children and their families seeking services, changes in healthcare coverage for families and a greater emphasis on providing preventive care. These societal factors remain relevant today.

Although tremendously efficacious and rewarding, group psychotherapy with children often leaves even seasoned group therapists feeling challenged. There are numerous resources that offer guidance with the technical aspects of children's groups. Child group therapists will find many quality handbooks, manuals and other resources filled with activities, games and handouts. While such resources are invaluable in working with children in groups, clinicians often find little of the theoretical richness that exists in approaches to adult group psychotherapy. Haen, writing in Haen and Aronson (2017), notes the paucity of research in the area of child group therapy. This lack of research is clearly a challenge faced by those working with children in groups. Further, there is far less theoretical richness found in the child group therapy literature than in that focused on adults. **Child group therapists are often burdened with the task of adapting theories developed with adults to their work with children. Clearly, a better grounding in a theoretical foundation is needed for our work with children in groups**. Those seeking to learn to work effectively with children in groups will be best served by an approach grounded in theory. Given the fact that much of the group psychotherapy theory available has been focused on adult work, the child group therapist is challenged with adapting that adult theory to work with children. It is a goal of the current book to assist the clinician with this endeavor.

This book offers the child group therapist a theoretical foundation that provides a meaningful framework to existing techniques. This theoretical foundation will guide the therapist, regardless of their level of experience or training. Although various

DOI: 10.4324/9781003189701-1

theoretical orientations are presented, **the primary foundation of the book is interpersonal group psychotherapy**. Regardless of the techniques and interventions employed and their theoretical origins, group work with children is most effective when it is highly interactional in nature. Child group therapy has always been rooted in experiential learning. Advances in our understanding of human brain development have supported the importance of interpersonal interaction and experiential learning. Yalom and Leszcz (2020), as well as Siegel (2020), underscore this in their books on group psychotherapy and brain development respectively. *Learning by doing is the most powerful approach with children*. Beebe and Lachmann (1994) note that the ongoing regulations that occur in the mother-child relationship help to organize the infant's experiences. Further, these authors propose that interactions with others in the environment continue to shape these experiences as children grow and develop. Children learn best through dynamic interactions that enhance the cognitive focus of a given group session. Whether through games, activities, role play, play therapy or other techniques, the interactive components of group therapy are where the power lies.

In seeking to bring a better theoretical foundation to group work with children, child development must serve as a guiding principle. Childhood is a dynamic time of change in all respects. The child group therapist must possess an awareness of the course of development in key areas. Such an awareness will often guide not only the types of interventions used but the ways in which they are delivered. Awareness of a child's developmental capacities allows the targeting of interventions at the optimal level for the best impact. **This book seeks to provide this awareness with a focus on three important areas of development: Cognitive, social/ interpersonal and intrapersonal**. These three areas are critical not only to a child's development but they are important focal points for our work with children in group therapy.

An interpersonal and highly interactional approach to group therapy assumes that a focus on group process is essential. Group process involves the experiences and examination of the here-and-now of the group – the emotional needs, wishes and fears manifested in the words and behaviors of the members Smead (1995), writing about the importance of a process focus in children's groups states, "Focusing on process, on the here-and-now, helps children learn to talk about immediate thoughts and feelings, which in turn may help them in their adult relationships" (p. 10). Brown (2003) refers to group process as the "here and now experience in the group that describes how the group is functioning, the quality of the relationships between and among the members and with the leader, the emotional experiences and reactions of the group, and the group's strongest desires and fears" (p. 228). Shechtman (2007) aptly states that children experiencing emotional difficulties "are not ready to be taught or trained in areas of skill deficit…" (p. 14). This author proposes that group therapy is most helpful when it allows the open expression of emotions in an intimate and empathic environment. Interventions solely focused on teaching and training on a cognitive level are not as effective. This book will guide the child group therapist in maximizing the potential of learning by doing and interacting with children. Schectman in Haen & Aronson (2017) names this approach "expressive supportive" (p. 52). The expressive supportive approach is characterized by the therapist engaging in critical behaviors that focus on support, information, clarification and attention to the ventilation of feelings (Shechtman, 2007, p. 17). Further, Shechtman (2007) notes that the therapist engages in "active listening, conveys concern and understanding, and thereby creates a holding environment" (p. 17). This approach does not preclude the use of more cognitively focused interventions such as psychoeducation, activities, and worksheets. It does, however, recognize that the true power of group therapy comes from here-and-now experience.

Group work with children poses challenges that often do not exist in adult groups. Primary among these is management of the child's behavior in the group. Too often, this is viewed from the standpoint purely of disciplinary action, isolated from the therapeutic process of the group itself. An interpersonal foundation to group work with children recasts behavior management as being an important and integral part of group process. Smead (1995) emphasizes the importance of using problem situations, such as disagreements or acting out, involving children's behaviors in the group as learning experiences (pp. 68, 69). Such a perspective brings this aspect of children's group therapy into the therapeutic milieu, and in doing so, greatly increases the power of the modality. Integration of interpersonal process work and behavior modification principles will offer the therapist a theoretically grounded approach to this often-challenging aspect of group therapy with children. **This manual will offer the group therapist practical recommendations regarding the management of behavior in the group room that comes from a process-oriented approach**.

This book seeks to infuse a multicultural and intersectional identity focus throughout. Considerable research in mental health as a discipline is foundationally WEIRD (White, educated, industrialized, rich and democratic). **It is essential to understand that many of the theories, techniques and interventions in group therapy, including those with children, were developed based upon a white-centric, heteronormative, cis-gendered, middle- and upper-class view**. In fact, many of the early developments in child group therapy occurred during a time in the United States when schools and other settings in which children operated were still racially segregated. Further, during the origins of group psychotherapy with children homosexuality was considered a mental illness and the continuum of gender identity was scarcely understood and not addressed. This book seeks to challenge the reader to better understand the potential impacts of these facts on diverse populations. We simply cannot assume that an understanding of group therapy based upon the majority view of the world will translate to the experience of all children and their families. **Therefore, this book will have as a core component challenges that guide the reader in thinking about issues of diversity and the experiences of those from marginalized groups**. Further, the book seeks to encourage and enable the group therapist in considering how their identity intersects with those of their clients.

Finally, this book will offer a systemic approach to groups with children that involves, to varying degrees, parents and others involved in a child's life (e.g. extended family members, teachers, coaches, case workers, other mental health professionals, medical professionals). Generalization of skills and interpersonal learning from the group room to other settings is an easily overlooked aspect of groups with children. **The book will emphasize the importance of communication with and involvement of parents and guardians in group work**. Two-way communication is the best way to ensure that work accomplished in the group generalizes to other settings (e.g. home, school, community). Two-way communication implies that there is input to the group therapist about the ongoing needs of the child and an outflow of information from the group therapist to collaterals allowing for the continuation of therapeutic work across settings.

The ultimate goal of this book is to offer the child group therapist, regardless of their level of training and experience, a unified approach to groups that is grounded in theory and available research. Most of the widely available resources for child group therapy are easily used within this framework. More specifically, this book seeks to offer a framework for utilizing games, activities and even treatment manuals in a way that still taps into the true power of group therapy, which is a process focus.

Group therapy with children represents some of the most challenging and rewarding work in the field of mental health. When considering the power of group therapy to improve the lives of children and their families, the reward is well worth the challenge. Group therapy has the power to transform the lives of children in many ways. Children who struggle with behavioral and emotional challenges often find a place where they belong in a therapeutic group setting. It is most rewarding to see children who might have felt like outsiders find relationships where they can begin to experience meaningful and gratifying connections with others. As these connections begin to produce changes in their emotional and behavioral health, it can be nothing short of miraculous.

History of Group Work with Children

The treatment of children in groups grew out of both necessity and observations about the natural tendencies of children to operate in groups. Schowalter (2003) notes the 1946 signing of the National Mental Health Act, the emergence of child guidance centers and the post war realization of the negative impacts of problems in childhood on adult functioning as factors in the child psychiatry movement. As psychiatry began to focus on the mental health needs of children, it is no surprise that group treatment became a predominant form of intervention. It has become widely accepted that children learn through experience. Arnett and Jensen (2019) stress the role of one's culture in development. It is through these interactions with others that we develop, particularly socially. After all, children are educated in classrooms that are, themselves, groups. From classrooms, to play groups, to birthday parties, children exist in groups. It is through the process of integrating the internal experience of children with the external reality of relationships that work with children progresses. Arnett and Jensen (2019) cite Margaret Mead noting that children progress from being 'lap children' from ages 0–2 years; to being 'knee children' from ages 3–4 years; and to being 'yard children' from ages 5–6 years. This progression from the lap to the yard so to speak exemplifies the ever-expanding social world of the child. It also serves as a metaphor for the increasing role played by interacting with peers in the 'yard' in socioemotional development.

Aronson in Haen & Aronson (2017) notes that "many early pioneers in the field of group work with youth had backgrounds as educators" (p. 2). Group therapy and education share a great deal of common ground. Group therapists and educators must be well-versed in child development. Further, they are focused on developing similar skills in children such as problem solving, interpersonal relationship capabilities and greater awareness of the self in the larger social context.

Group therapy developed out of the need to serve more children in a setting that was natural for them. Further, as with adults, groups permitted the serving of more people in an efficient manner. Multiple children could be served in a relatively short period of time. Over the course of time, multiple theories of group have emerged. Some of these will be reviewed as a means of offering the reader an overview of different approaches.

Psychoanalytic Approach to Groups

Samuel R. Slavson, the founder of the American Group Psychotherapy Association (AGPA), was a proponent of progressive education and the child guidance movement. He did extensive work with children in the early-to-mid 20th century. He defined group therapy as "an aggregation of three or more persons in an informal face to face relation, in direct and dynamic interaction with one another" (Slavson, 1979, p. 524). Further, Slavson posed the concept of social hunger, defined as "a need and the capacity for object relations and group acceptance." He believed that this was a prerequisite for inclusion in a therapy group.

Slavson engaged children in Activity Group Therapy (AGT), which involved creating a "permissive environment" in which children could express emotions and develop autonomy. In the early stages of the group, the child can use the environment in whatever way they wish. Slavson (1979) writes that the child "can make friends or withdraw, work or idle, construct or break, quarrel, fight or fraternize" (p. 546). Activity Group Therapy groups placed six to eight latency-aged children in a specially equipped room (with age-appropriate toys and games) in which they are free to act out their impulses, "as aggressive as they may be" (p. 546). A trained therapist observes the group and intervenes as needed, primarily around "practical circumstances related to the children's work and play and maintenance of the meeting room" (Schiffer, in Riester & Kraft, 1986, p. 233). The therapist was careful with their interventions in order to avoid influencing the direction of the group or responding in ways that might be typical of other adults in the child's life. "Out of the chaos emerges a degree of order within the children and the integration of their psychic forces" (p. 574). This leads to what Slavson called

> Activity Catharsis where children work out their frustrations using toys in the therapeutic environment. Members have responsibility for the structure and function of the group. The leader only responds when called upon. The leader reacts in a manner unlike any other adult.
>
> (p. 549)

This can involve any of the following:

1   Choosing to ignore the behavior or
2   Providing some interpretation to clarify the behavior.

This minimal involvement is focused on "not usurp(ing) the patients' ego and superego functions" (p. 542).

Activity Group Therapy certainly runs counter to modern ways of intervening with children in groups. While ignoring of some behaviors is used as an intervention in children's groups, this does not occur to the degree that it did in Activity Group Therapy. Further, the long-term nature of Activity Group Therapy (often a minimum of two years) would certainly not fit all settings in the current healthcare environment.

Similarly, Riester and Kraft (1986) note that Bender reported using group therapy to treat children in a hospital ward in the 1930s. They go on to state that early attempts at treating children in groups "engaged children in learning through experience and activity" (p. 4). These authors further note that these early uses of group to treat children employed both "the progressive education premise that children learn from here-and-now experience" and "the psychoanalytic assumption that experience and peer interactions can 'work through' conflicts and self-barricades in a nonverbal medium" (p. 4). Anna Freud emphasized the importance of the child's interactions with family members and other groups in which they operate (Altman et al., 2002; Riester & Kraft, 1986). These ideas continue to underlie much of the child group therapy that is conducted today. Recent brain research has supported some of these key ideas from a psychoanalytic approach to groups.

Obviously, these approaches to group therapy with children, particularly Activity Group Therapy, anchor the more non-directive end of the spectrum with regard to leadership. It is widely accepted today that Activity Group Therapy in its pure form is contraindicated (Schiffer, in Riester & Kraft, 1986). This is due to a number of factors including patient safety, time constraints of modern treatments and the general recognition that the therapist must take a more active role in the treatment of children in their groups.

An archived video of Mortimer Schiffer (who worked with Slavson) conducting an Activity Therapy group demonstrates how this model existed in a different time from our own. The video shows a group of middle-school-aged boys who are white and likely from middle and upper middle-class backgrounds playing with tools (hammers, drills, saws, etc.) in a room. There is minimal supervision of these youth, and they are permitted to work out whatever impulses they might have with the provided tools. Despite this more permissive and arguably dangerous environment, this model does inform us that overly directive forms of group therapy with children can be of equally dubious value. There is a happy medium between the permissive environment and the more controlled and directive classroom type approach that is employed in more structured settings, thereby losing some of the process focus. Finding this happy medium allows for group process and for what Shechtman calls the expressive supportive environment to develop.

Counseling Groups

A second school of thought emerges out of the educational counseling field. Mariane Schneider Corey, Gerald Corey and Cindy Corey (2018) describe an Integrative Approach to group therapy. These authors use a Thinking, Feeling and Behaving Model that takes into account these three components of a client's experience of the group. They write, "Combining these three domains is the basis for a powerful and comprehensive approach to counseling practice" (p. 103).

Corey et al. (2018) outline a variety of types of groups within the counseling framework that is based upon those defined by the Association for Specialists in Group Work (ASGW). While the Coreys work primarily with adults, their definitions of the types of groups are helpful in understanding the evolution of child group therapy.

Many groups with children incorporate elements of each of these types of groups. When we speak of group psychotherapy with children, we are typically referring to groups that fall into the categories of counseling and psychotherapy groups. However, there are also task groups, psychoeducational groups and even brief group therapy models that are conducted with children. The focus of this manual will be on the categories of counseling and psychotherapy groups with children.

Rosemarie Smead (1995) adapted the work of the Coreys to children in some really important ways. As with the Coreys, her work is based upon a "Thinking, Feeling, Behaving" model (p. 135) that is largely based on a Cognitive Behavioral approach and psychoeducation(?). Smead proposes that these three dimensions of experience are central to effective work with children. She defines these as follows:

- **Thinking** – "…all the cognitive processes that take place in the mind: recollecting, comprehending, analyzing, synthesizing, creating, imagining, reasoning, reflecting, judging, forming opinions and beliefs, and valuing" (p. 135).
- **Feelings** – "are complex events having both cognitive and physiological components… these are the result of our appraisal of a situation as either positive or negative" (p. 135).

Group Type	Purpose	Examples
Task Groups	Application of group dynamics principles and processes to improve practice and to foster accomplishment of identified work goals (p.7)	Learning groups, school groups, discussion groups, study circles (p.7)
Psychoeducational Groups	Developing members' cognitive, affective, and behavioral skills through a structured set of procedures within and across group meetings (p.7)	Anger management groups, Communication and social skills groups, friendship groups, bullying prevention groups (p.8)
Counseling Groups	Focus on interpersonal and problem-solving strategies that stress conscious thoughts, feelings, and behavior (p.9)	Groups that assist members in developing more positive attitudes and better interpersonal skills; use group process to facilitate behavior change; help members transfer newly acquired skills and behavior outside the group (p.9)
Psychotherapy Groups	Help individual group members remediate psychological problems and interpersonal problems of living (p.10)	Groups that focus on deeper and more significant psychological disturbance; alleviation of symptoms of a disorder (p.10-11)
Brief Group Therapy	Groups that are time-limited, have a preset time for termination (p.11)	More structured groups that incorporate characteristics of both counseling and psychoeducational groups (p.11)

Figure 1.1 Corey's Group Types

- **Behaving** – "includes both overt actions (e.g. throwing a ball, reciting a poem, getting into an argument) and covert actions (e.g. a heartbeat or having a headache" (p. 135).

Smead suggests that the purposes of the group are to (1) teach children to monitor their thoughts, replacing negative ones with positive ones; (2) help children identify their own feelings and develop empathy for others' emotional experiences and (3) develop positive behaviors. Replacing negative thoughts with positive ones might involve changing thoughts such as 'I'm a bad kid' to 'I'm a good kid.' Positive behaviors might include adaptive ways of dealing with bullying, saying 'no' to peer pressure or communicating one's needs more directly to those in one's life.

While there is great value in this approach to group therapy, there is a risk of focusing too much on the individual, thereby missing some of the powerful dynamics that go on interpersonally. If groups are overly focused on the individual member and very structured, much of the power of the modality is lost. There are two dimensions that deserve particular attention by the group therapist. These are (1) the degree to which the focus is on the individual vs. the group and (2) the degree to which there is focus on the structure of the group vs. group process. As will be discussed in later Chapters, the degree of structure in a group varies depending on many variables. Likewise, there are varying degrees of focus on the individual versus the group dynamics.

Cognitive Behavioral Group Therapy

Christner and Bernstein in Haen & Aronson (2017) note that Cognitive Behavioral Therapy (CBT) "suggests that an individual's thoughts mediate his or her emotions and behavioral responses to certain situations and events…" (p.111). CBT considers how thoughts, emotions and behaviors work together to impact a child's decisions and actions. Christner and Bernstein note a core set of techniques that are used in CBT with children (pp. 114–119):

- Psychoeducation
- Cognitive Restructuring
- Relaxation Training
- Role Play and Practice
- Teaching Problem-Solving Skills
- Homework
- Planning for Generalization and Maintenance of Behaviors and Skills outside the group setting

CBT has as a foundational tenet that if a person's thoughts are changed, their emotions and behavior will change as well (Corey et al., 2018). Many of the aforementioned techniques have broad applicability with children and the teaching of skills, role play and planning for generalization are often-used techniques in all groups regardless of their primary theoretical orientation.

The child group therapist is reminded, however, that these techniques are best employed with a here-and-now process-oriented focus. Further, with CBT approaches, there can be a great deal of emphasis on psychoeducation and the individual instead of on the group. It is important to bear in mind that a process focus has been shown to truly capture the dynamics of group therapy. These approaches are best used when there is a learning by doing approach. For example, the teaching of problem-solving skills can be done in a very active manner using role play of real-life problems with the group-as-a-whole. This engages more learning modalities and brings the cognitive aspects of situations to life in the group room.

Interpersonal Group Psychotherapy

Yalom and Leszcz (2020) have developed the interpersonal theory of group psychotherapy. This approach takes a here-and-now, process-oriented approach to groups. **The interpersonal approach to group psychotherapy considers the experiencing and exploring of interactions among group members to be the primary mechanism of change for members of the group**. These authors identified 11 therapeutic factors in group therapy that are key aspects of the modality. These are (p. 10):

- Instillation of Hope
- Universality
- Imparting Information
- Altruism
- Corrective recapitulation of the primary family group
- Development of Socializing Techniques
- Imitative Behavior
- Interpersonal Learning

- Group Cohesiveness
- Catharsis
- Existential Factors

Shechtman (2007) and Sheppard (2008) have explored the adaptation of these therapeutic factors and other aspects of the interpersonal approach to work with children. Additionally, Corder et al. (1981) found that the therapeutic factors adults find most relevant are similar to those endorsed by adolescents. Because it is so foundational to interpersonal work with children, this will be explored further in subsequent Chapters of this manual.

Smead (1995), referencing the work of Yalom and Leszcz (2020), differentiates between *content* and *process* in children's groups. Content is defined as "…what members are talking about, the subject of the present conversation" (p. 9). She notes that content usually has a "there-and-then" focus, typically from the group room both spatially and temporally as when a group member discusses a trip to the zoo or a troubling occurrence in their classroom. In contrast, process focuses on exploring and understanding "…the nature of the relationships among the group members who are communicating with one another" (p. 9). Process usually has a "here-and-now" focus. For example, in the above example, a process focus examines how the event is unfolding within the group. Perhaps members are not really listening to the speaker or the speaker is not attending to the others and doesn't realize that they are bored or lost. Smead (1995), Corey et al. (2018), Yalom and Leszcz (2020) and many other influential voices in the field have established the power of a "here-and-now" focus in groups. This is true not only of adult groups, but of children's groups. Manualized and overly cognitive approaches to children's groups can take on too much of a "there-and-then focus" losing the power of the "here-and-now" experience of the child. Yalom and Leszcz state, "When the therapy group focuses on the here-and-now, it increases in power and effectiveness" (p. 49). This could not be more true of children's groups and will be a major focus on this book.

It is noted that interventions from other approaches such as CBT can be employed in the context of an interpersonal approach. From a developmental perspective, children are not capable of pure process-oriented group work where the focus is on verbally processing occurrences in the group. Therefore, it is strongly recommended that children's groups include a balance between content and process.

Group as a Powerful Modality in the Treatment of Children

It has been established that group is a powerful modality in working with children. Aronson (2017) notes that "the field of child and adolescent group therapy has experienced tremendous growth" since its inception (p. 4). Further, he states, "groups are now rightly seen as a powerful format for providing help and support for youth facing a wide range of challenges so they can proceed with the developmental tasks ahead" (p. 4). Group therapy offers help with a number of challenges faced by today's children. The list below includes some of these challenges that are frequently addressed in group therapy:

- Depression
- Anxiety
- Behavioral Problems
- Impulse Control Problems
- Attention Deficit Hyperactivity Disorder (ADHD)

- Low Self-Esteem
- Divorce of Parents/Blended Family Concerns
- Social Skills Deficits
- Anger Control
- Attachment Disorders
- Trauma
- Relational Issues

While this list is nowhere close to exhaustive, it does provide the reader with a sampling of some of the many issues that are frequently addressed in group settings. Beyond this list of frequently addressed challenges, there are some issues faced by children that are actually best addressed in a group setting. Some of these presenting issues have a significant relational component where interpersonal learning and the ability to practice skills with other children are critical. Other issues are amenable to group therapy due to the active nature of the modality. For example, depressed children often benefit from the activating effects of a group setting. **The following list presents some specific presenting issues that are often best addressed in group therapy**:

- Attention Deficit Hyperactivity Disorder (ADHD)
- Relational Issues
- Autism Spectrum Disorders
- Interpersonal/Communication Delays
- Impulse Control Disorders
- Depression
- Behavioral Disorders
- Anxiety Disorders

Integration of the Dynamic and Cognitive in Child Group Therapy: Interpersonal Neurobiology

The field of Interpersonal Neurobiology (IPNB) based upon the work of Daniel Seigel has given us a framework for understanding the way human relationships impact brain development. Gantt and Badenoch (2013) write,

> an awareness of IPNB principles might put a firmer foundation underneath us as group leaders so that we can approach our groups with greater awareness of how to contain the group and develop the group's capacity to support the neurobiological changes that underlie richer relationships.
>
> (p. xvi)

This is applicable to child group therapy in that it provides brain-based explanations for many of the processes that have been accepted for years. Those working with children in groups are intervening at a critical time in brain and relationship development. An awareness that relational input shapes the brain is an idea that puts group therapy at the forefront of interventions for children. This is due to the aforementioned interactive nature of group therapy. In therapy groups, children are able to learn and practice skills in a social environment, thereby increasing the likelihood of their being integrated into their repertoire of coping, interpersonal and self-management capacities. Further, children learn how to better interact with adult group leaders and co-leaders. This, in turn, helps them to navigate relationships with other adults in a more adaptive manner.

Interpersonal neurobiology suggests that a more targeted and integrated approach is critical. It also offers a framework for accomplishing this integration. Current neurobiological research has emphasized the interpersonal nature of human brain development. Numerous authors including Siegel (2020) and Badenoch and Cox (2010) have written about the role of implicit memory in learning and development. Implicit memory is highly experiential in nature. There is a "felt experience" quality to it. Tapping into this in children's groups through highly experiential learning is of the utmost importance in capturing the full power of group therapy. Experiential learning for children is often described as "learning by doing." For example, this might include talking children through the steps of solving an interpersonal problem as they are doing it or shortly thereafter. There are important implications for the ways that human beings learn in IPNB:

*   The emphasis is shifted away from talking and more exclusively cognitive interventions.
*   The focus is placed upon *experiential learning* through interpersonal process.

For example, from an interpersonal neurobiology perspective, there is more value in role-playing anger situations with children or even coaching them through an anger episode than a strictly psychoeducational approach that "teaches" steps to anger management. Even more effective might be an intervention that teaches steps to anger management through role play and application to real-life situations. Combining the cognitive and the experiential maximizes the intervention.

Siegel (2020) states "…human connections shape neural connections and each contributes to mind. Relationships and neural linkages together shape the mind." (p. 7). This supports the use of group therapy, which is at its very core a social modality. It emphasizes the focus on interventions and techniques that utilize interpersonal interaction and group process. It suggests that the interaction surrounding purely cognitive activities (worksheets, games, puzzles, etc.) is critical to therapeutic change. The child group therapy literature is rich with techniques, activities and interventions, which can be used to facilitate the integration of interpersonal interaction with a more cognitive approach. **Regardless of the techniques employed and their theoretical origins, group work with children is most effective when its primary focus is on human interaction**. The group therapist is reminded that if the focus is solely on these interventions (worksheets, activities, games, etc.) much of the power of group therapy is lost.

Clinical Vignette

The following clinical vignette is intended to introduce the reader to an interpersonal, process-oriented focus with children. In this vignette, it is the first session of a group for depressed and anxious children. The group consists of six members in 4th and 5th grades of diverse backgrounds and two group leaders. In this particular interaction, members are asked to introduce themselves to the group. They have been provided with a list of things to share about themselves that includes the following:

*   My Name
*   My School

- My Grade
- Pets I have or had
- A food I like to eat
- Something I like to do/My Hobby
- Something I like about this group so far

During the introductions, one of the co-leaders is taking notes as members introduce themselves. To encourage listening and paying attention to each other, this leader will engage the members in a "quiz" where they can earn points for answering correctly questions such as "Who in our group likes to eat popcorn?" One of the group co-leaders volunteers to go first with introductions so that members have a model for how to do their introduction and thus help manage anxiety in the group. This vignette picks up after the co-leader's introduction.

GROUP LEADER 1: "OK, so we heard from Dr. Z. Who would like to go next with their introduction?"

SUSAN: "I will. I'll go next."

GROUP LEADER 1: "OK, Susan, that would be great."

SUSAN: "My name is Susan and I go to the West End Academy and I'm in 4th grade. I have a dog named Bill and I had a fish named Ted, but he died…"

As Susan is talking, Group Leader 2 notices that two members are whispering to each other.

GROUP LEADER 2: "Trey and Lincoln, I noticed you were whispering to each other while Susan was talking. Remember to pay attention so that you'll be able to earn some points in our quiz later."

Both Trey and Lincoln apologize and get into a listening posture. Susan finishes her introduction.

SUSAN: "…I like to eat pizza and I like to collect Pokémon cards. Something I like about this group so far is that the teachers are nice."

TREY: "I'll go next. My name is Trey and I go to South Lake Elementary and I'm in 5th grade. I don't have any pets because my parents are allergic to animals."

SAMMI: "Wait. What? You don't have any pets? Does that make you sad?"

TREY: "Not really. I've never really thought about it."

SAMMI: "I would be so sad if I didn't have my dog, Honey. She's my best friend. I like taking her to the park for runs and to play frisbee. The other day, she caught the frisbee five times in a row!!"

GROUP LEADER 2: "Sammi, I'm really glad to hear about your dog and how you'd be sad if you didn't have her, but I think you interrupted Trey while he was doing his introduction."

SAMMI: "OK. Sorry about that."

GROUP LEADER 2: "It's OK. We're all learning how group is going to work. And I guess we might all be a little nervous with group being new to us right now. Sammi you were trying to connect with Trey wondering if he might be sad, as you would be, if you didn't have a pet. Is that right?"

SAMMI: "Yeah. That's right."

GROUP LEADER 2: "I like that you were curious about how Trey might be feeling. In group it's a good thing to ask about others' feelings. Let's find a way to do that that doesn't interrupt what others are saying. Maybe for now we could get back to our introductions. Trey, I think you were going to tell us about a food you like to eat."

Trey continues his introduction.

TREY: "…I like to eat pizza and I play the guitar. Something I like about this group so far is that the chairs are comfy."

As introductions progress, the group leaders are linking group members by emphasizing things that they have in common. For example, they might point out that three members are in 4th grade and three are in 5th grade. They might also point out that two members don't have pets. This is a way of beginning to form connections in the group and to build cohesion, which will be discussed in detail later in this manual.

Group Leader 2: "I just noticed that both Trey and Susan like to eat pizza. That is something that the two of you have in common."

In this vignette, the group leaders are attempting to foster a "here-and-now" focus in the group. The quiz is meant to introduce the expectation of being present in the "here-and-now" by listening and attending to others as they introduce themselves. The leaders also attempted to balance group process with content. This occurred when there was an interruption by Sammi while Trey was talking. The group leader wants to honor the curiosity about another group member's feelings (process) while maintaining the focus on the activity at hand (content). The group leaders will guide the group in finding ways to be curious about each other but to do this in a way that follows the rules and guidelines of the group (e.g., one person talks at a time).

Summary

Group psychotherapy is a powerful tool in the treatment of children. Many issues and challenges that are faced by today's children are amenable to being addressed in a group setting. There are a number of theoretical approaches to group work with children. Further, the group therapy literature is quite robust with activities, worksheets, games and other interventions for use with children. The child group therapist is reminded that these are most effective when used in the context of a here-and-now, process-oriented approach.

This book seeks to guide the clinician in considering essential knowledge and skills that are needed to successfully build and orchestrate effective therapy groups for children. This work will serve as a 'best-practices' manual for the child group therapist. Further, it will emphasize diversity, child development, the importance of play, the integration of theory and practice and practical matters facing the group therapist.

The book is divided into eight chapters, each focusing on a different aspect of group psychotherapy with children. These chapters are listed below along with their page numbers for ease of reference.

Structure of the Book

Chapter 1-Foundations of Group Psychotherapy with Children
Chapter 2-Child Development for the Group Therapist
Chapter 3-Multiculturalism for Child Group Therapy
Chapter 4-Interpersonal Theoretical Foundations
Chapter 5-Therapist Considerations
Chapter 6-Group Development
Chapter 7-Ethical Considerations in Child Group Therapy
Chapter 8-Practical Matters in Child Group Therapy

Each of these chapters will include vignettes and case examples that illustrate the principles covered. These examples are meant to assist the child group therapist in developing the necessary knowledge, attitudes and skills to build and facilitate successful therapy groups with children. Some chapters contain critical thinking activities that allow the reader to think critically and to reflect upon concepts covered. Each chapter has clinical vignettes and activities tailored to the specific content. Whether this book is used for self-study or taught in a group format, these questions and activities are meant to spur thought and discussion about the concepts that are presented.

Questions for Discussion and Review

1   Consider how to integrate activities (e.g., worksheets, games) and group process in a children's group. Discuss the balance between the cognitive and the interactive.
2   Consider the benefits and limitations of Slavson's Activity Group Therapy (AGT). How would a modern clinician take elements of this approach and use them today?
3   Consider elements of the five types of groups presented that would be helpful in designing a children's therapy group. How could components of each enhance effectiveness?
4   Discuss the benefits and limitations of treating various presenting issues with children in a group setting.
5   Discuss the power of experiential learning in children's groups. Consider examples of how this can be employed with different presenting problems.

Exercise

A Multicultural Perspective on Theory

The Association for Specialists in Group Work (ASGW) has developed a set of strategies that seek to address issues related to equity, multiculturalism and social justice in groups. Guth et al. (2019) state the importance of "acknowledging that dynamics of both culture and power are inherent in any group setting" (p. 8). Further, they encourage group workers to "be mindful that upon first contact they enter into a relationship with group members that is nestled within the constructs of co-mingling cultural identities and power structures" (p. 8). It is critical that we consider this in our work with clients.

As mentioned previously in this Chapter, many theories of group psychotherapy were developed by white individuals based upon their work with predominantly white middle-class clients. The following critical thinking activity asks the learner to consider this and other issues surrounding culture and identity. The American Counseling Association (ACA) Multicultural and Social Justice Counseling Competencies (Ratts et al., 2016) encourage group therapists to consider the issues of counselor self-awareness and client worldview as critical parts of developing multicultural competence.

The ASGW (2019) strategies recommend cultivation of cultural humility. This is defined as seeking to "humbly understand how cultural identity shapes the worldview and experiences of others" (p. 16). These authors encourage group therapists to "learn about themselves through an intersectional cultural lens" (p. 16).

Questions for Thought and Discussion

•   How is the self-awareness of the group therapist impacted by theory? What is the impact of this on multicultural awareness? What implicit biases exist in the theories we are taught?
•   How do we best align ourselves with the client's worldview? How do we listen most effectively to our client's experience of the world, especially those different from our own? What are the signs that we are imposing our worldview on our client?

   o   Consider these identities that children might bring into group:
      ▪   Other than straight sexual orientation

- Other than cis-gender identity
- Children of same-sex parents
- BIPOC (Black Indigenous and Persons of Color) identified children
- Immigrant children
- Children of immigrant parents
- Multi-racial children
- Adopted children
- Children with differing levels of ability
  ○ How might these identities and their potential intersectionality impact their worldview?

References

Altman, N., Briggs, R., Frankel, J., Gensler, D., & Pantone, P. (2002). *Relational child psychotherapy*. New York: Other Press.

Arnett, J. J., & Jensen, L. A. (2019). *Human development: A cultural approach*. New York: Pearson Education.

Badenoch, B., & Cox, P. (2010). Integrating interpersonal neurobiology with group psychotherapy. *International Journal of Group Psychotherapy, 60*(4), 462–481. https://doi.org/10.1521/ijgp.2010.60.4.462

Beebe, B., and Frank M. L. Representation and internalization in infancy: Three principles of salience. *Relational Psychoanalysis, 2*, 227–274. https://doi.org/10.4324/9780203728062-14

Brown, N. (2003). Conceptualizing process. *International Journal of Group Psychotherapy, 53*(2), 225–244. https://doi.org/10.1521/ijgp.53.2.225.42814

Corder, B. F., Whiteside, L., & Haizlip, T. M. (1981). A study of curative factors in group psychotherapy with adolescents. *International Journal of Group Psychotherapy, 31*(3), 345–354. https://doi.org/10.1080/00207284.1981.11491712

Corey, C., Corey, G., & Corey, M. S. (2018). *Groups: Process and practice*. Boston, MA: Cengage Learning.

Gant, S. P., & Badenoch, B. (Eds.). (2013). *The interpersonal neurobiology of group psychotherapy and group process*. London: Karnac Books.

Guth, L. J., Nitza, A., Pollard, B. L., Puig, A., Chan, C. D., Bailey, H., & Singh, A. A. (2019). Ten Strategies to intentionally use group work to transform hate, facilitate courageous conversations, and enhance community building. *The Journal for Specialists in Group Work, 44*(1), 3–24.

Haen, C., & Aronson, S. (2017). *Handbook of Child and Adolescent Group therapy: A practitioner's reference* (pp. 193–202). New York: Routledge.

Kratochwill, T. R., & Stoiber, K. C. (1998). *Handbook of group intervention for children and families*. Boston, MA: Allyn and Bacon.

Ratts, M. J., Singh, A. A., Nassar-McMillan, S., Butler, S. K., & McCullough, J. R. (2016). Multicultural and social justice counseling competencies: Guidelines for the counseling profession. *Journal of Multicultural Counseling and Development, 44*(1), 28–48. https://doi.org/10.1002/jmcd.12035

Riester, A. E., & Kraft, I. A. (1986). *Child group psychotherapy: Future tense*. Madison, CT: International Universities Press.

Schaefer, C. E. (1999). *Short-term psychotherapy groups for children: Adapting group processes for specific problems*. Northvale, NJ: J. Aronson.

Schowalter, J. E., MD. (2003). A history of child and adolescent psychiatry in the United States [Abstract]. *Psychiatric Times, 20*(9), 9th ser.

Shechtman, Z. (2007). *Group counseling and psychotherapy with children and adolescents: Theory, Research, and Practice*. New York: Routledge.

Sheppard, T. L. (2008). *Group psychotherapy with children*. New York: American Group Psychotherapy Association.

Siegel, D. J. (2020). *The developing mind: How relationships and the brain interact to shape who we are.* New York: Guilford Press.

Slavson, S. R. (1979). *Dynamics of group psychotherapy: Ed. in consultation with the author by Mortimer Schiffer.* London: Aronson.

Smead, R. (1995). *Skills and techniques for group work with children and adolescents.* Champaign, IL: Research Press.

Yalom, I. D., & Leszcz, M. (2020). *The theory and practice of group psychotherapy.* New York: Basic Books.

2 Child Development for the Group Psychotherapist

Zachary J. Thieneman

Introduction

Understanding human development is of critical importance to the child therapist. The complex, multilayered constructs of child development impact each member's ability to interact with the group and vastly alter the effectiveness of interventions. Awareness of the ways in which children develop is essential in working effectively with them. In her book *The Child Therapist*, Brems (1994) emphasizes the importance of training in child development for any therapist wishing to work with children. Among the areas that Brems suggests must be covered are "specific developmental aspects such as cognition, psychosocial…motor and language development…" (p. 11). In order to effectively work as a child group therapist, you must first understand the intricacies of development – and where your clients land in the vast spectrum of human maturation.

Therapeutic or educational work with children must consider the fact that they are 'works in progress.' Contrary to myths from early in psychology's history, children are not 'little adults.' Their worlds and brains mature over time and are capable of different cognitive and interpersonal tasks based on their point in development. It is now understood brain maturation extends well into young adulthood (Johnson et al., 2009; Sowell et al., 1999). Unlike adults, with whom neurological development is considered somewhat static, children are dynamically growing in regard to their cognitive, social and intrapersonal abilities. This chapter seeks to address interpersonal process work and how development impacts groups by overviewing prominent theories and how development can influence children's ability to engage with group tasks.

The extra layer of development onto child groups makes them exceptionally challenging. The need for the child group therapist to possess knowledge of development is multitudinous with three overarching points guiding this chapter.

1 **Development guides goodness of fit for a specific child in a specific group**. The child group therapist must be capable of determining the developmental "level" of a current or presenting client to understand their functional capacity. Tailoring groups to a child's "level" incorporates all aspects of a child's current maturation and uses this information to guide goodness of fit. Many groups have gone awry from disparate composition of members all over the developmental spectrum. Have you ever tried to run a group with both teenagers and preschoolers? While possible, their points in development necessitate different needs and teenagers would be better suited to a group with teenagers. Age, like social, cognitive and emotional maturity, are broad markers for a child's goodness of fit in a group. The same goes for school-age children – have you ever tried running

DOI: 10.4324/9781003189701-2

a group with emotionally mature and emotionally immature preschoolers? While similar age, emotionally mature preschoolers require different interventions than preschoolers with little regulatory skills. Too much variability between group members can lead groups astray because of the difference of interventions required. Creating effective child groups requires an understanding of development to ensure the clients entering the group have the highest chance of success. A group similar enough in intellectual functioning, social functioning and emotional regulation, just like in adult groups, allows the group to form and work together. With children, similar development facilitates group cohesion and is vital to the success of child groups.

2   **Development guides interventions in child groups**. By understanding a child's individual maturation, the child group therapist is more likely to style interventions in a way which maps onto client needs and thus greater success. A child's point-in-time development will impact their interaction with and response to interventions in the group. Targeting one's interventions to a child's individual developmental level across experiential realms (e.g., cognitive, emotional, interpersonal) is an often-overlooked factor in the success of interventions. Schamess (as cited in Riester & Kraft, 1986) states, "I have seen far too many talented therapists leave the field after excruciating experiences in which they attempted to use a treatment model that did not recognize the members' developmental needs…" (p. 33). The field of child group therapy has lost many talented clinicians failing to take a developmental perspective. The use of developmental models to guide our assessment of and intervention with children ensures maximum effectiveness in group therapy. Slavson (as cited in Riester & Kraft, 1986, p. 9), stated: "If the child is to grow into a balanced adult, the natural movement from dependence needs to be encouraged and so canalized as to strengthen his character." The ultimate goal of the therapy group is to put the child on a developmental trajectory that will lead to healthy functioning in subsequent stages of life. Doing so requires tailoring interventions based on each child group's developmental tasks. Throughout this chapter, overarching theories provide helpful avenues for styling interventions.

3   **Development is not monolithic**. The world of development is heavily influenced by majority views in American research culture. Many theories do not take into account views of those outside the majority culture. For example, Piaget's theory does not take into account people with intellectual differences; attachment theory does not include worldwide anthropology and the myriad routes to healthy attachment; Bandura's famous Bobo Doll study (Bandura, 1965), an integral study supporting Social Learning Theory, involved participants attending the privileged Stanford University nursery.

Most major developmental theories involve white, middle-upper class samples. Much behavioral science research comes from a specific population, and one that is WEIRD: Western, Educated, Industrialized, Rich and Democratic (Henrich et al., 2010). It is imperative that broader social and cultural contexts are taken into account when making universal developmental implications. Swanson et al. (2003) said it best when discussing models for racial and ethnic minority youth developmental research: "Too often empirical investigations do not address the interactive effects of structural conditions, historical forces, psychological processes, and a priori assumptions of psychopathology" (p. 767). Development is not monolithic; rather, it is a rich, complex, human tapestry deeply intertwined to culture and individual characteristics.

In order to decolonize psychological history, theory shortcomings must be addressed in current treatment with clients to honor and use individual and cultural variations to maximize treatment outcomes. **Multicultural considerations *must* be overlayed onto**

theory to best understand our clients' worlds and create best practices. Given the complexity of human development, there is no overarching theory which represents everything. The theories discussed in this chapter are launching pads for understanding in greater detail the universality of human experiences which may vastly differ from culture to culture, in known and unknown ways. Miller (2011) advocates looking at various theories to integrate them into a holistic picture. This author describes developmental theories as having three tasks:

(1) to *describe* changes *within* one or several areas of behavior,
(2) to *describe* changes in the relations *among* several areas of behavior, and
(3) to *explain* the course of development that has been described.

(p. 8)

This work will present models of development in three key realms closely related to child group therapy: Cognitive; interpersonal/social; and intrapersonal. Although each area of development is highly interactive with the others, it is useful to discuss each in isolation, how they relate to one another and how they directly impact child groups. It is important to note that each section is a highly condensed version of the represented content and should be treated as a brief overview applied directly to child groups.

Several prominent theories have structured and shaped the conversation about human development into our current understanding. Many of these theories have since expanded, revised and changed over time to account for the vast differences in global human behavior. The following theoretical models will be presented for consideration:

- Piaget's Cognitive Development (Piaget & Inhelder, 1969)
- Information Processing Theory (Miller, 1956)
- Social Learning Theory (Bandura, 1977)
- Socio-Cultural Theory (Vygotsky, 1978)
- Attachment Theory (Bowlby, 1958)

Theories are starting points and should be considered as such. The more we understand about development, the more questions we ask. Many questions remain about the universality of developmental experiences. Best practice means clinicians contextualize and conceptualize development within the individual frameworks of their clients.

Case Example

Throughout this chapter, a case example of a children's therapy group will be used to exemplify critical theory components. Below is a brief introduction to the group:

- **Jamal**, eight-year-old Black, cisgender male diagnosed with Reactive Attachment Disorder and oppositional defiant disorder;
- **Jasmine**, nine-year-old Black, cisgender female diagnosed with Social Anxiety;
- **Harry**, seven-year-old White, cisgender male diagnosed with Attention-Deficit/Hyperactivity Disorder and an Unspecified Depressive Disorder;
- **Hawa**, eight-year-old Latinx, cisgender female diagnosed with Generalized Anxiety;
- **George**, seven-year-old White, cisgender male diagnosed with Autism Spectrum, Level One, Without Intellectual Impairment;

- **Jimmy**, an eight-year-old Latinx, cisgender male diagnosed with Disruptive Mood Dysregulation Disorder with a rule-out for Posttraumatic Stress Disorder;
- The group leader is a cisgender, White male in his 50s with a PhD in Counseling Psychology from a middle socioeconomic status. He is native to the United States.

Human development encompasses an incredible amount of information. As you read this chapter, consider your clients and child groups while thinking critically about the areas of human development you know well and those areas with which you could further develop your understanding. Think about how you might modify your group processes and interventions based on application of developmental theories!

Cognitive Development

Long understood to be the vessel of childhood learning, play is known to be vital to all aspects of a child's development. Children experience, explore and learn through play. This was known to Piaget, one of the pioneering cognitive psychologists of the 20th century. Piaget's Theory of Cognitive Development shaped and continues to shape conversations about how cognition matures over time. Play is a cognitive process through which children learn – and an avenue to style group interventions with children. Cognitive development may seem unrelated to child group therapy at times due to its basis in cognitive neuroscience. Child cognition is directly applicable to child groups when initially creating a child group, identifying goodness of fit for a new member, applying interventions to children at different ages and different levels of maturation and processing efficacy of interventions. In fact, tailoring interventions using a developmental perspective is vital to successful child and adolescent therapy (Garber et al., 2016; Kinney, 1991; Oles, 1991).

- **Piaget's Theory of Cognitive Development** is a discontinuous, stage-wise theory which starts at infancy and continues through early adolescence. Many of the constructs within Piaget's theory are at least in part consistent with current neurological research, though Piaget himself struggled with the stage-wise nature of his own theory which did not account for individual differences and cannot universally encompass development.
- **Information Processing Theory** helps fill in some of the gaps in Piaget's theory by focusing on the process, not the stage or content, of continual cognitive development.

First and foremost, childhood cognition builds upon itself. Much like a complex array of LEGOs®, cognitive tasks build upon each other to form new and composite images. Therefore, if a deficit exists at one stage, it may continue to influence subsequent stages of development. Piaget and Inhelder (1969) stated, "if the child partly explains the adult, it can also be said that each period of his development partly explains the period that follows" (p. 3).

Cognition is similar in some ways to language. Language develops over time and uses increasingly larger vocabulary to describe minute nuances. Words like the Indonesian 'mencolek,' which means to tap someone on their opposite shoulder to get them to look the wrong way, are highly relative to specific cultures. Just like native English-speakers would likely not know this word, children may not understand complex ideas such as "emotional regulation."

Language, like cognition, is inherently tied to children's ability to engage with therapeutic interventions. **Cognitive theories provide guideposts for interventions so clinicians can meet the clients where they are and provide best practices for children**.

Piaget's Theory of Cognitive Development

As stated previously, *development is not monolithic*. Different cognitive skills are emphasized in different cultures around the world. In our groups, we must attend to the individual cognitive skills of our child clients to ensure they accurately comprehend group messages. Piaget's Cognitive Development provides a structure of cognitive tasks crucial for the child group leader to understand in order to design interventions and assess member fit when considering group composition.

Piaget's initial stages (without sub-stages as they are beyond the scope of this book):

- Sensorimotor Stage
- Preoperational Stage
- Concrete Operational Stage
- Formal Operational Stage

Sensorimotor Stage. The sensorimotor stage normally occurs roughly from birth to two years. This stage is preverbal where children explore the world using physical, sensory interactions which provide cause-and-effect learning. During this time, infants learn basic cognitive tasks which are the precursors to language and memory. Infants and toddlers, from a development perspective, are setting the cognitive stage for more complexity as they age. Object permanence, for example, is the idea that once an object leaves an infant's line of site, it continues to exist. While this is obvious to an adult, very young children are still learning basic cognitive tasks which slowly expand and build upon each other over time. Interestingly enough, infants are very social beings with natural pulls towards caregivers. Beatrice Beebe and Daniel Stern offer a moment-by-moment analytic view of mother-infant dyads they refer to as *microanalysis* (Beebe, 2017). Microanalysis looks at videotaped, brief, moment-by-moment interactions between an infant and mother and how they influence each other. As it turns out, Stern (1971) found mother-infant communication is:

- co-created by the unique dyad,
- bidirectional communication,
- co-regulatory.

Beebe and Stern's work implicates the co-regulatory nature of relationships throughout the lifespan, including infants. Even during infancy, children are social beings communicating and learning in their social environments! Stern's body of work directly relates to the co-regulatory nature of therapy and the overall impact of relationships *starting in infancy*. However, it is unlikely group therapists will encounter many participants at this age!

Preoperational Stage. The preoperational stage normally emerges approximately from two years to seven years old. During this time, major cognitive tasks include the emergence of language, basic representational thought and perspective-taking. Piaget and Inhelder (1969) describe representational thought as "the ability to represent something…by means of a signifier which is differentiated and which serves only a representative purpose: language, mental image, symbolic gesture, and so on" (p. 51). Children at this stage are egocentric, rigid thinkers who experience the world in semi-logical ways (often referred to as "kid logic") and do not generalize effectively. Magical thinking is a great example. Children who dress up as certain characters might believe them to be those characters, or if they dress like them enough they will become the character! The playfulness inherent in preoperational thinking is exactly why play activities are crucial during this stage. Play-focused therapy allows clinicians to effect change while working within the mental constructs through which children at this age experience the world.

Children at this stage require interventions which are

- **concrete,**
- **playful,**
- **focused and**
- **directly relevant to their experience.**

Group therapists working with this age range focus on play activities that are concrete, directly observable experiences which promote a specific learning goal. Too much abstract language may be difficult to comprehend. A concrete play activity is an action-oriented activity with ties to the here and now which has some form of physical representation, often of a more complex idea. For example, "positivity basketball" can be used to promote supportive ties between group members. Using a real or made-up basket, members are encouraged to create a fake "trick shot" and on-looking members are given the task of making positive statements to the member taking the shot. This takes an abstract idea, being positive to others in group, and turns it into a concrete play activity. Play takes many forms: A group-wide game, a turn-taking activity, show-and-tell, dyadic LEGO®-building or role-playing using puppets to name a few.

Let's take emotional language as the content of a group activity. Many children need practice regulating their emotions – starting with recognizing emotions in themselves and others. If we apply the concepts of preoperational cognitive development onto the childhood task of emotional regulation, one possible outcome is playing emotions charades. Emotions charades is exactly as it sounds, with the group as a whole guessing one member's various emotional expressions. Emotions charades allows children to play pretend while relying on their lived experience within their families and cultures of origin. Instead of talking about emotions, they are playing emotions by acting them out and guessing the feeling. A game like emotions charades is a useful strategy to help children in the stage of preoperational cognitive development to begin to identify various emotions in themselves and others. Experiential learning is vital as it links direct experience to positive, novel scenarios. Imagine the following interaction between two group members while playing emotions charades:

GROUP LEADER (QUIETLY TO GEORGE): "Alright, George. Can you show us anger?"

GEORGE: "Okay." (George stands up and balls his fists but remains expressionless on his face)

JIMMY: "He looks, like, sleepy. Are you sleepy, George?"

GEORGE: "I'm not sleepy! My parents get mad like this!" (George continues to ball his fists while sitting and remaining expressionless)

GROUP LEADER: "It sounds like you all talk about and act out anger in different ways. Jimmy, can you show us what anger looks like for you?"

JIMMY: "Sure! It looks like THIS: CÁLLATE! GET IN YOUR ROOM NOW!" (Jimmy shouts, balls his fist, puffs out his chest and holds his breath to make his face red)

GROUP LEADER: "Wow – your anger is not like George's anger. Did you notice? (Jimmy and George nod). What is the difference between the two?"

JIMMY: "George's anger was sleepy. Mine was ANGRY." (Jimmy nods slowly while saying his last word)

GEORGE: "Jimmy yelled and his face got really red and he was stomping around really loud. Jimmy's anger was a BLOWUP. BLOWUPS are bad. I get in trouble when I BLOWUP. I would lose Fortnite FOREVER if I did that."

JIMMY: "My anger isn't bad! I'll show YOU a BLOWUP!" (Jimmy stands up)

GROUP LEADER, STANDING UP: "Hold on a second, Jimmy! Let's take a break. Do you think you could sit down while we take our break? (Jimmy stares at George then turns away from him and sits down) Thank you, Jimmy. Can we all take five big, slow breaths?" (group practices breathing exercise) You all rock!

"Our families teach us lots of different things, don't they? People show feelings individually. Jimmy and George, you have two separate experiences with anger, and both are awesome, just like you. Feelings, just like how we show them, are neither right nor wrong. We are responsible for our actions when we have big feelings like anger, but it is always okay to feel! I appreciate you showing the group what anger looks like, both of you showed excellent examples. Tell me more about anger in your families…"

Children need to *learn by doing*. Learning by doing with play and activities is vital to child comprehension and well-documented for different populations (González-González, 2021; Önder, 2018; Perrier, 2004). In the example above, George and Jimmy exemplified emotional expressions seen in their families of origin. They might, along with the rest of the group, be asked to show different family members in their house being angry and how they calm down afterwards. In an example such as this one, anger expressions are exemplified based on cultures of origin. Different cultures encourage disparate emotional expression based on values and identity statuses (Cole et al., 2006; Okur & Corapci, 2016).

Note the therapeutic response from the group clinician which doesn't identify a "right" way to express emotions. Clients enter into therapy with varying messages related to emotions which can be shared and talked about as a group to enrich overall knowledge rather than focus on the "wrong" way to express feelings. The example also differentiates emotional experience vs. emotional expression and actions. This difference is crucial to the childhood understanding of emotions which are often emotional experience, emotional expression and actions tied into one! By differentiating these aspects of emotions, children are also encouraged to be responsible for their actions and emotional expressions while experiencing high emotions.

The social microcosm seen in adult groups is ever-present in child groups with peer-to-peer learning stemming from concrete member experiences. Games like emotions charades are a means of creating healthy, fun, applied learning environments which "play" to the developmental strengths of children!

Children can color, interact with peers, engage in dyadic conversation and have a concrete visualization of an abstract idea. Instead of setting goals verbally, children can draw a treasure map which details exactly how they are going to achieve their goals and steps along the way. All of these ideas, like emotions charades or treasure maps, are tailored to the developmental tasks of the children's ages. An activity such as treasure maps concretizes an otherwise abstract concept while naturally targeting developmental tasks such as perspective-taking (e.g., "What did your moms say you should work on in group?"). In other words, it turns into *learning by doing*. Even Mr. Rogers in his famous neighborhood understood the importance of play. He agreed with Piaget that play is serious learning for children!

Concrete Operational Stage. The concrete operational stage is normally from ages 7–11 years old. During this stage comes the emergence of increasingly complex mental operations. Major learning feats include temporal awareness, advanced cause and effect, abstract thought such as interpersonal relationships and self-esteem, autonomy, linking bodily experiences to cognitive experiences, generalization of rules and basic organization of a sense of self. These tasks show up in child groups with examples like perspective-taking, reading emotions of other group members, attending to how an individual's actions impact others in the group, noticing how emotional expression and actions are related to internal emotional experiences, or using group rules in other settings such as school. Like the preoperational stage, experiential learning continues to benefit concrete operational children with an emphasis on generalizing to novel situations. Budding complexity allows for more advanced and distinct topics which incorporate all of the aspects of working with children previously discussed: **Activity, play and peer-to-peer interactions remain excellent ways to design interventions and build group cohesion during the concrete operational stage**.

Many children enter group treatment at this stage with the onset of increasing environmental demands like school, socialization and home expectations. As children's worlds are becoming more complex, so can group interventions. Emotional language is a good example. Many children are able to identify the base emotion of sadness. Adults by comparison might have ten different words for sad and articulate nuanced distinctions in their expression. The concrete operational stage is a developmental stage where children's internal worlds vastly expand and cognitive sophistication allows for deeper connection. Instead of one word (sad) they might develop gradations such as "down" or "depressed" while discovering triggers for each.

Simply talking about feelings is a difficult (and often boring) task for children. Consider the following activity for developing a deeper understanding of sadness: Emotions target. After some psychoeducation, children are asked to throw a sticky hand or ball at a target. The target has gradations of sadness written on individual rings: Down, gloomy, sad, sorrowful and depressed. Oftentimes, this is in the context of how each feeling relates to thoughts, actions and bodily sensations in order to pair internal and external experiences. When each member has their turn, they practice talking about the specific ring they hit and a time when they felt that specific feeling. Group members watching are encouraged to verbally support the member who is tossing. If time allows, they may even construct a scene showcasing the target feeling word from their home and identify members to help them act it out!

Think about how this activity relates to concrete operational thinking. Emotions target is

- playful,
- action-oriented,
- encourages deepening abstraction and complexity and
- allows for peer-to-peer interaction.

In other words, an activity like emotions target effectively tailors an abstract intervention (emotion-focused psychoeducation) in a kid-friendly, concrete, playful activity.

Imagine taking emotions target to the next level. Concrete operational children are beginning to learn complex ideas. Level two of emotions target could overlay several feelings on the emotions target in order to describe the experience of multiple feelings at the same time! Imagine splitting your concrete operational group into dyads. Each group could practice simultaneously in pairs or have an example dyad at the front to showcase the skill. Each dyad then has to have one member be the "sculptor" and one member be the "sculpture." Sculptors have to use language to describe what a certain combination of feelings looks like on each sculpture. Sculptures have to follow the sculptor directions and freeze in place. The group then comes together and shows off each "sculpture." Consider the following case example:

GROUP LEADER: "Alright, Jasmine and George, you all will be working together to help 'sculpt' some emotions, just like we did with anger and anxiety. To start, we need a pair to show the group what we are doing. We are going to practice 'sculpting' sadness. Jasmine, you did such an awesome job listening while we were talking about anger. Would you like to be the sculptor or the sculpted?"

JASMINE: "I want to be the sculptor!" (Jasmine shows visible excitement)

GEORGE: (Stands up and walks over to Jasmine) "Fiiiiiiine. Can I go next?"

GROUP LEADER: Remember, just like the last time we practiced sculpting emotions, everybody will get a turn. George, can you start by showing us sadness?"

GEORGE: (stands up and lowers his head but remains expressionless in his face) "There."

JIMMY: "Why does George look sleepy again?"

GROUP LEADER: "It sounds like what you are saying is that George's angry and sad look similar. Is that correct, Jimmy? (Jimmy nods) Alright, do you all notice this as well? (Most of the group nods) Okay, I see what you mean. George, are you ready for some sculpting? (George nods) Go for it, Jasmine!"

JASMINE: (moves in to touch George's face) "Can you move your…"

GEORGE: (swats Jasmine's hand and backs away) "DON'T TOUCH ME, YOU KNOW I DON'T LIKE TO BE TOUCHED!" (Jasmine freezes and looks extremely anxious)

GROUP LEADER: "Accidents happen, and you don't like to be touched, I remember this from the last time we played. I am wondering if this happens again could you can ask calmly and back away instead of hitting Jasmine's hand? (George nods. Thank you. Jasmine, are you able to continue? I can see you look anxious. (Jasmine does not move or respond and several seconds go by in silence). Jasmine, it is okay to feel anxious. Would you like to take a moment to unfreeze? I bet one of our friends in group can help you finish sculpting. Who would you like to help you? (Several more seconds go by and Jasmine points to Hawa). Thanks, Jasmine! I know how hard it is to unfreeze and you did such a great job choosing. Hawa, would you like to help? (Hawa nods) Great! Switch places with Jasmine, then. (Jasmine sits down and Hawa stands up). Hawa, thanks for helping Jasmine. That was very kind of you. Remember, George does not like to be touched. Can you use your words and help George show us sadness?"

Hawa, pausing for a moment to think and look at George: "George, move your shoulders down like THIS? (lowers shoulders to a slumping posture, George mirrors) Make your eyes look down, too. (Hawa lowers her eyes to look at the floor then takes a few moments to think). I don't know what else."

GROUP LEADER: "Great suggestions, Hawa. Does anybody have any other ideas?"

Jasmine, raising her hand quickly: "Can he put his lip out, like this?" (Jasmine puffs out her bottom lip)

GROUP LEADER: "Nice idea! Let's see it, George!" (George sticks out his bottom lip, just a little)

Jasmine (waits a few seconds looking at George): "MORE George, like THIS." (Jasmine sticks out her bottom lip in an exaggerated way, and George mirrors) Yeah!"

GROUP LEADER: "Okay friends, does this look like sad to you? (most of the group nods) Now that you have an idea, let's all split up and practice showing each other what sadness looks like for you…"

Using play and activities encourages concretization through '**learning by doing**.' Abstract, internal experiences can be effectively targeted using concrete, external activities. An activity like sculpting helps children articulate their experiences and express their emotions. This plays to the strengths of concrete operational children who are developing concepts of abstraction and extrapolation.

Creativity is often a part of play. Clinicians need to remain flexible and creative while thinking about the content in order to apply it to their child group. Like the sculpture and emotions target activities, playful interventions overlay aspects of development onto specific content to create a focus for the group. **Groups require different activities suited to the children who comprise them**. We may not do an activity with a physical target when members have been exposed to gun violence or a sculpture activity with children who have experienced trauma (sometimes while sculpting children may invade personal space while trying to articulate what they want the "sculpture" to do). The point is to use creativity to enhance and expand play activities with each unique group. Doing so enriches and enlivens the experience for children and leaders.

Formal Operation Stage. The last stage Piaget theorized is the formal operation stage, from ages 11 to 15. While this stage moves from childhood into adolescence, it is important for group therapists to actively use the cognitive development of their active stage to prepare them for effective functioning in subsequent stages of development, in this case moving from the concrete thinking of younger ages to the increasingly abstract world of adult thought. Formal operational thought involves what Miller (2011) defines as thought that has become "truly logical, abstract, and hypothetical" (p. 57). Thinking at this stage is largely differentiated by:

- Abstract thinking
- Creativity
- Hypothetical reasoning
- Hypothesis-testing

While thought was previously tied to concrete experiences and direct observation, children at this age develop abstract understanding of the world around them. For example, children and teens at this age understand the scientific method and advanced cause-and-effect to see the impact of their actions on others more so than younger children. If a 14-year-old makes a microaggression in group, they may readily interpret the impact of those words on other members, making this age a great place to practice perspective-taking and advanced feelings exploration.

Interestingly enough, children and teens at this age understand advanced theoretical topics such as physics but do not always think logically. They may evidence hypothetical reasoning in physics and get an 'A' in the class but might say something mean in an argument with their mother and not foresee the consequences!

Think about the differences between clients in adolescence and younger children. Imagine you have one group of formal operational thinkers who are 13–15 years old. Your other group is our case example in this Chapter, all seven to nine years old. Imagine both groups experience religion-based microaggressions. For example, a member experiences a microaggression related to their Islamic faith from a Christian member. You decide to practice a perspective-taking activity in each group. The same microaggression and the same intervention are planned but the group members are at vastly different points in development. Think about the following:

- How would you design perspective-taking activities for each group?
- What would be different?
- What would be similar?

The cognitive sophistication, logical deductions, generalization of skills and thought organization markedly increase with age. In the formal operation stage, youth between 13 and 15 years old are capable of more routine "talk therapy" but may still enjoy playful interactions and interventions which are sophisticated echoes of their childhood. In a perspective-taking activity, it is likely the formal operations group can talk through cause and effect of the microaggressions with less scaffolding. They could articulate feeling hurt, offended or stereotyped by those words. The clear cause and effect is present and a repair can be made by educating the group verbally about harmful stereotypes and how they negatively impact others.

However, talking through microaggressions would be considerably tougher for the younger, preoperational children seven to nine years old. Considering cognitive development, the perspective-taking activity needs to be modified and mapped onto their development. One method would be to physically take the perspectives of others or "putting yourself in their shoes." By literally role reversing and encouraging members to think outside of their own selves, they can see in concrete ways how stereotypes are harmful to others and feel hurtful. In both cases, asking the aggressor to imagine being the target of the microaggression is a method to handle the situation during group but needs to be done with sensitivity to cognitive development.

Postformal Thought. Piaget's theory has been continually revised and expanded with new research particularly from the fields of neuroscience and evolutionary biology, such as the idea of postformal thought which seeks to identify how brain maturation carries forward into adolescence and adulthood (Scott-Janda & Karakok, 2016). Piaget's stages are largely considered an underestimation of cognitive abilities. Neo-Piagetian theorists posit children are capable of learning more, and quicker, than Piaget originally theorized.

Postformal thinking includes more sophisticated cognitive processes such as dialectics and *thinking about thinking* (Scott-Janda & Karakok, 2016). Cognitive development does not simply end in teens as Piaget initially thought, but becomes increasingly more complex. Research continues to illuminate what this complex thinking entails and how it may be further studied, such as the many different ways people may solve a singular problem without the need for a right or wrong distinction (Cartwright et al., 2009).

The predominant point of postformal thought expands upon the limitations of Piaget's theory and how, even as adolescents and young adults, we continue to grow. Piaget's theory launched a world of investigation into the differences within human cognitive development and outlined the importance of cognition when working with children. One lasting aspect is the idea of a growth mindset when working with children. **Growth mindset is vital to child group therapists: Viewing our clients through the lens of development provides a window into the child world and challenges us to apply interventions that best fit their developmental level**.

Exercise

Think about your current groups or a group you plan to create. Where are your clients within the general framework provided by Piaget's Theory of Cognitive Development? What is one play activity you might create using the basic cognitive learning tasks of the Concrete Operational Stage?

Information Processing Theory

As our tools for research and brain monitoring increase, so does our body of knowledge relative to cognition. Considerable research exists in neuroscience and evolutionary neurobiology which provide rich understanding of cognitive development. For example, Piaget fought with the concepts of continuity and discontinuity within his work, struggling to identify exactly when and how children may move from one cognitive stage to the next (Bibace, 2013). This is where theories such as Information Processing are exceptionally helpful as they fill in the idea of continuity and *how* humans learn information. Information Processing Theory is a cognitive theory directly applicable to group interventions. Understanding how children learn in the moment is valuable for child group therapists to:

- Identify the cognitive mechanisms underlying group content to ensure retention;
- Identify signs of attention and inattention during group;
- Actively style interventions in the here-and-now of the child group;
- Process efficacy of interventions across time based on client application of group content.

Information Processing Theory uses computers as a metaphor for the human brain, identifying various structures and their impact on behavior, thought and learning. Information Processing

Theory has changed significantly in recent years, originally comparing human brains to computers while also noting the incredible complexity of the brain and how that differentiates it from any modern computer (Ashcraft, 2009). While different from Piaget's model, information processing offers a complimentary viewpoint of human development. First and foremost, information processing is a continuous approach rather than a stage-wise, discontinuous model as Piaget suggested. Information Processing Theory identifies the in-the-moment cognitive processes governing the learning of a new concept. This continuous approach, making the assumption that human brains are constantly and steadily growing, marks an important point in the fluidity of human development – the individual differences between same-age peers. While Piaget provides a broad estimation of cognitive tasks of developing children spanning years, information processing examines the here-and-now learning.

Information Processing Theory has several basic assumptions:

- information moves through a series of cognitive processes within an individual (attention, perception, short-term memory, long-term memory);
- processing transforms information as it is encoded, such as interpreting visual stimuli into meaningful mental objects (e.g. recognizing a red octagon on the street as a STOP sign);
- the more a stimuli is attended to, the more likely it is to be encoded into short-term memory and then into long-term memory, especially with repeated rehearsal and
- understanding these processes involves understanding underlying brain structures as one might understand pieces of a computer working together for an output. **While focused on memory and the cognitive processing of information, Information Processing Theory has vast implications for effective child group therapy**.

Information Processing and "Brain Breaks." In the world of child group therapy, understanding developmental theories is integral to application of interventions and evaluation of their success (and failure). As we begin to understand the *how* of the developing mind, we also learn *how* to apply clinical interventions developmentally with our specific clients and *how* to process with children. Sometimes a "brain break" can be an important tool during child groups. Sustained attention is challenging for most adults, let alone developing minds. This is even more true if you are running a group after school! Child clinicians must therefore flexibly approach clients and their ability to sustain attention (or not) by creating space for literal breaks to reset attention regulation processes. Sometimes child clients simply need to "get the wiggles out" before a structured activity! Realistically, children's limited capacity for sustained attention impacts anything you do in group sessions.

Imagine you are running a group for younger children ages four to six in an outpatient practice. You are working on introducing a new member who joined this session. The group sat patiently as everybody introduced themselves. After the introductions are finished, you notice they are starting to seem restless. You have to correct several of them to attend to the activity at hand, but it's not working and most members continue to appear aloof. You have a really neat activity which should be fun, but requires them to pay attention. Do you continue with the session as planned or not?

In the above clinical scenario, which is a very common occurrence in child groups, the group leader could choose to continue the activity. The activity might appear to be successful, but at the same time pursuing the activity also negates appreciating the feedback the group is providing the group leader: *They aren't ready to focus right now.* The intervention as a whole is not likely to be attended to, received, rehearsed or encoded into memory! A different route which tailors to development and may help promote sustained attention is taking a "brain break."

As a group leader, you decide the members just aren't ready to learn through your activity at this exact moment. You find your remote control (an old remote for a CD player which nobody uses) and hit "pause" on the group. The group freezes and you tell them you notice they need a break. The group nods and you take a break. After a few minutes, the group seems to calm down. They are able to sit and redirect their attention back to you as the leader. You ask the group if they are now ready to play a game and press "play" before proceeding with the planned activity.

Child clinicians must attend to the feedback from the group, which isn't always verbal. With younger children, they are more likely to act out their experiences than speak to them. Group leaders therefore must monitor the group's verbal and non-verbal messages throughout a session as a means of feedback to flexibly meet the group's needs. The younger the average age of the group, the more important and frequent become. Children can handle very limited amounts of directly clinical activities. Groups with members who struggle with attention regulation need even *more* breaks on average.

Allowing time for "brain breaks" also works to our cognitive advantage: It ensures members are ready to perceive and understand our message for the day. From the example above, you could even use the remote to pause, play, rewind or fast-forward group or individual members as a method to process group interactions!

Brain and movement breaks provide built-in "pause" buttons for the group which can be used for process work. In this way, we practice moving from the attention level of encoding to the perception level outlined in Information Processing Theory. Whenever a group is struggling to attend to group content, there is an opportunity to hit "pause." The group could then take a break to play a short movement game or fun mindfulness activity. Before returning to the group content, it is possible to bring the attentional difficulty into the here and now by talking about it via questions such as:

- "I noticed as a group we are having a hard time focusing today. Tell me about it!"
- "Is this something you all experience all the time, like at school?"
- "How do you know when you need to take a break like we just did?"
- "How does your body and mind feel after our break? How did they feel before the break? What's different between the two?"

Think about it this way: By pressing the "pause" button during group to process moments with members, even preoperational-age children, we give them the ability to modify their thinking for future interactions, develop intrapersonal awareness and develop regulatory skills! This is all done through understanding how children learn and noticing it during child group sessions. **By looking at how children learn, we are also teaching ourselves as clinicians to decipher process work with children**. Attending to cognitive readiness and the engagement of a child group directly allows clinicians to 'slow down' an activity which is akin to making process comments in adult groups. Many adult clinicians are surprised to learn how important process work is with children. Process-level work simply looks different with children than with adults but remains vital to the success of the group. Social cognition is an integral part of both the change process and cognitive development. In fact, repeated process work threaded through content allows members to directly relate their internal experience to the broader group experience and provides a vessel for feedback. Process work with children leads to an internalization of those experiences and can act as a "shot of positivity."

Information Processing Theory encourages us to look closely at how we engage with our members and underscores the challenges of an adult clinician working with children. Child group work is similar to translating a message–except from one language to another, it is from one point in development to another. Clinicians must translate their knowledge into a developmentally appropriate message. **Working with children necessitates we communicate in a way which is both clinically relevant and kid-friendly**. Information Processing Theory teaches us to look more closely at the behaviors of our child groups to ensure they are ready to learn.

Discussion Questions

1   How does cognitive development impact interventions for group therapy with children? How might it impact group cohesion?
2   Think for a moment about Piaget's cognitive development model and how it relates to group psychotherapy with children. How might you design a relaxation intervention for anxiety with children who are five and six years old vs. children who are 10 and 11?
3   Imagine parent involvement in the group. How might parent involvement be different with younger children in the preoperational stage vs. children who are teenagers in the formal operational stage?
4   How do you work with people who have intellectual disabilities within your practice? What adjustments might you make for a client who has an intellectual disability and is a good fit for one of your groups?

Social/Interpersonal Development

"Through others, we become ourselves." L.S. Vygotsky (1987)

Healthy relationships are palliative by their very nature. This is the heart and power of any therapy group and broader still, any mode of psychotherapy. Contrary to previous thinking where a child's cognitive development was considered to limit socialization, in reality children at all developmental levels are **social, dynamic, relational beings**. In fact, relational skills are crucial to neurological development (Bjorklund, 2018). Recent research indicates how much the brains of children are constantly discovering, observing and learning about the world around them. During toddler-hood, children gain new synapses in the prefrontal cortex at a rate of 2 million *per second* (Shonkoff & Phillips, 2000)!

Neuroscience research indicates children are highly open to interpersonal input which will form functional social foundations throughout life. For example, children benefit from sibling relationships when processing parent, academic and peer-related issues (Brody, 2004). As described earlier through Beebe and Stern's work, even infants have the capacities and desires to engage in and help regulate social interactions! More than ever, we understand how interpersonal interaction impacts brain development and, thereby, the parameters for coping, learning and growth.

Humans have the astounding ability to learn from and within changing environments – children are no exception. Socialization is one of the most important tasks of childhood. Development of socializing techniques and interpersonal learning are vital therapeutic factors of group according to Yalom and Leszcz (2020). As such, this makes group therapy an effective modality for the emerging mind as it allows for and directly facilitates social learning. During therapy groups, children learn through interactions with peers and the healing relationships within groups.

Using the vast amount of research on social development and learning, major theories offer key insights into effective child group psychotherapy. Bandura, Erikson and Vygotsky were some of the pioneering, classic developmental theorists who initiated decades of research on socialization. Modern critiques of these theories overlay culture onto social development to illustrate one of the main points of this chapter: **Development is *not* monolithic but dynamic and richly varied**.

In the following sections, we discuss Bandura's Social Learning Theory, Erikson's Psychosocial Stages of Development and Vygotsky's Sociocultural Theory, more specifically, the Zone of Proximal Development. **Like cognitive development, social development stems from other branches of behavioral sciences crucial for the child group therapist to understand and apply with child groups**.

Social Learning Theory

Bandura's Social Learning Theory was an incredibly impactful theory at its inception in the 1970s and still holds merit to this day, albeit in more complex forms. Social Learning Theory built on Skinnerian behavioral models emphasizing reinforcement and its impact on human behavior. **Bandura posited people learn vicariously through those around them, most especially peers**. Likeness of models leads to enhanced learning (Rodriguez Buritica et al., 2016), though children receive and learn through social messages in their everyday environment from both adults and peers.

Children learn to imitate and imitate to learn (Zmyj & Seehagen, 2013): Children watching violent television are more likely to be violent; children who witness healthy group norms are likely to engage in healthy group behavior; children on a playground learn to play from their peers. Imitative learning has vast implications for group therapy with children. We know healthy groups have strong, supportive interpersonal dynamics which lead to group cohesion. Group cohesion is well-documented to be one of the most meaningful aspects of groups. **Tying group cohesion and social learning together, we have a built-in vessel for understanding how to build a healthy group climate with children**. A healthy group climate is a safe launch pad for child members to explore psychosocial difficulties.

One of Bandura's primary building blocks and tenets of social learning is the idea of **vicarious reinforcement**: "new behaviors can be acquired simply by watching a model who is reinforced" (Miller, 2011, p. 234). This basic premise of vicarious reinforcement holds true today. For example, if a child in group is *not* reinforced for making a mean comment while another child is reinforced for a positive comment towards a group member, the group will have an opportunity to learn that making nice comments will lead to positive reinforcement. Over time, and possibly outside of their conscious awareness, children learn such social lessons through basic group processes such as maintaining group norms. Here's another clinical example to illustrate the idea of vicarious reinforcement:

A child in your group, Brandon, routinely feels distracted and unable to attend to the group activity. He repeatedly seeks attention of the leaders, specific members or the group as a whole. After discussion with your co-leader, you decide to ignore Brandon and encourage the group members to do the same. You decide to talk to the group so you can strategize how to handle the situation. You and your co-leader provide stickers to other members who ignore Brandon when he is acting out while you withhold stickers for Brandon until he engages with the group activity. Surprisingly, the group is able to ignore Brandon for the first half of the session while he attempts various ways to get their attention. Over the course of the session, however, Brandon starts to engage with the group activity and is then reinforced for this new social engagement. By the end of the session, Brandon has helped another group member draw a picture, which was part of the activity!

Paired with the efficacy of external rewards for children (as opposed to adults), interventions using vicarious reinforcement have far-reaching implications for the development of group cohesion. **By strategically processing interactions and encouraging healthy**

exchanges, we are providing group-as-a-whole interventions even if we are only addressing two members. It is important to note that reinforcement can also inadvertently support 'bad' behavior as when a leader provides increased attention to an acting out child which can then encourage other children to act out.

Due to **observational learning**, or acquiring behaviors based on observed reinforced or non-reinforced models, group leaders must be keenly aware of the behaviors reinforced, not reinforced and punished within their groups. Examples of actions which are often unintentionally reinforced include:

- unhealthy attention-seeking,
- scapegoating,
- monopolizing,
- bragging about negative behaviors,
- stonewalling,
- criticisms,
- aggressive behavior,
- dishonesty and
- interruptions.

Disruptive behaviors have the potential to derail child groups. Sometimes, members are so disruptive they demand interventions which can reinforce the behavior and thus teach it to other members. Understanding vicarious reinforcement, observational learning and their downsides allows for creative solutions which do not inadvertently increase problematic group behaviors.

Reinforcing positive behaviors such as

- honest sharing of feelings,
- following group rules,
- compassion,
- inclusion of members,
- perspective-taking,
- healthy coping skills,
- pro-social behaviors (validating, active listening, empathy) and
- in-vivo use of group skills

encourages group cohesion and safety which are foundational to successful groups.

Social cognition teaches the value of group norms that encourage healthy relational functioning. In turn, healthy relational functioning contributes to the healing power of group. Imagine the group is learning about various expressions for similar emotions and acting out feelings on a feelings thermometer. In this group, participants earn stickers for participating in group activities and following group rules. Think about the following scenario from the sample group:

GROUP LEADER: "You all did such a nice job talking about feelings for our thermometer. I gave Hawa an extra sticker for telling us so many good words for anxiety and Harry an additional sticker for paying attention. Harry, I know how hard it is for you to sit still when we talk about things like feeling thermometers. I appreciated that you showed me your whole listening body by making eye contact, not interrupting and sitting up in your seat while we talked. Nice work! Hawa, since you did such an amazing job with giving us different words for anxiety, how about you be the first one to act out a feeling? (Hawa stands up and walks to the middle of the room) Thanks, Hawa! You jumped right in, that's great. We have to try and guess which word it is. Can you whisper to me what word you are acting out so I know as well? If you need help, look at the board which has our words listed: worried, concerned, anxious, preoccupied, nervous, uneasy, fearful and PANIC. (Hawa whispers she is going to show panic) Go for it, Hawa!"

HAWA: "AUGH!" (Hawa yells and puts her arms over her head, flailing them around while running in circles and then hiding behind a chair. The group laughs as Hawa runs around. As Hawa hides behind the chair, the group quiets down)

GROUP LEADER: "Hawa, thank you. Any guesses?"

GEORGE: (raises hand quickly) "Anxious!"

GROUP LEADER: "That's very possible. I like how closely you were watching Hawa when she was acting. Any other guesses?"

HARRY: (raises hand) "I think it was PANIC. She was, like, freaking out and acting all weird."

GROUP LEADER: "Those are both great guesses. Any others? (Nobody raises their hand) Hawa, what was it?"

HAWA: "PANIC!" (Hawa returns back to her seat)

GROUP LEADER: "Harry, how did you know it was panic and not one of our other anxiety words?"

HARRY: "She, like, raised her arms around and hid. Her eyes were really big and she screamed. (Harry raises his arms and makes a face imitating Hawa's panic demonstration) That's like a big feeling. Panic's a REALLY big feeling."

GROUP LEADER: "You're right! Panic is a big feeling. It's at the top of our anxiety thermometer. It's very different than, say, nervous where people don't usually flail their arms around like that. George, do you see the difference? (George nods slowly) I am going to give the entire group a sticker for listening and watching so carefully. Jamal, I really liked how you were using your listening body to give Hawa your attention. Hawa, you did an excellent job demonstrating. I am going to give you an extra sticker for showing the group what panic looks like for you. Harry, I am also giving you an extra sticker for showing us some things to pay attention to when we are acting out emotions!"

Think about all of the observational learning and vicarious reinforcement that occurred in the example above. The entire interaction would have taken no more than one to two minutes! Right at the beginning, both Hawa and Harry were reinforced for engaging appropriately with the emotions activity. Even though they were not directly involved, George, Jimmy, Jasmine and Jamal all can learn through Hawa and Harry's vicarious reinforcement that following group rules and norms is rewarded in group. As these external rewards also influence member's internal representations of themselves, members begin to internalize they are "good kids." The specific, labeled praise of the group leader is also instructive to the rest of the group who were not involved in the interaction. Think about George's interpretation of Hawa's panic. Even though he did not guess the emotion Hawa was showing, other members of the group learned that it is okay to guess incorrectly and participate in activities without fear of being right or wrong. With so many opportunities for observational learning in each session, it is no small wonder how powerful group interventions can be for the developing social mind!

Stages of Psychosocial Development

Erik Erikson's Stages of Psychosocial Development provide a framework for establishing the primary psychosocial task of a given age. This stage theory, like Piaget's, posits psychosocial developmental tasks for a given age range. In Erikson's theory, issues from various stages may not be fully resolved and children can become stuck in particular tasks. Furthermore, each stage's tasks are framed as dichotomous outcomes. For example, without a basic sense of safety, children may be mistrustful of others. Group therapy brings to light unresolved issues and provides an avenue for corrective experiences based on individual client needs. Furthermore, groups may be *conceptualized and characterized* using Erikson's stages while progressing through group and individual tasks over the group's lifespan. In other words, the group as a whole can be seen as moving through the developmental stages of Erikson's psychosocial development. For the purposes of a child focus, only the stages until puberty will be discussed in greater depth (Figure 2.1).

Stage	Age Range (Estimated)	Tasks
Trust vs. Mistrust	Birth- Two years	Attachment, Hope
Autonomy vs. Shame and Doubt	One-and-a-half to three years	Will, security
Initiative vs. Guilt	Three-five years	Purpose, budding initiative
Industry vs. Inferiority	Six-11 years	Competence, expectations, accomplishments
Identity vs. Confusion	12-18 years	Fidelity, peer relationships, identification
Intimacy vs. Isolation	19-40 years	Love, deeper relationships
Generativity vs. Stagnation	40-65 years	Care, engagement with younger generations
Integrity vs. Despair	65-death	Wisdom, life accomplishments, reflections

Figure 2.1 Erikson's Stages of Psychosocial Development

Erikson (1950) stated the first task, basic trust is: "the infant's first social achievement, then, is his willingness to let the mother out of sight without undue anxiety or rage, because she has become an inner certainty as well as an outer predictability." (p. 247). Other theorists identified similar processes including Mahler's separation-individuation and Bowlby's attachment theories which both focus on infant social relationships (for a comparison, see Bergman et al., 2015). Infants' social worlds often encompass family members, friends and community others who are caregiving. Safety for young children stems from familiarity with those whom they interact and the predictability of their environment. Many children presenting for group therapy may not have a basic sense of security due to their life circumstances. Groups offer security and emotional safety which are vital to their success. Providing and working through basic safety facilitates growth through this stage of psychosocial development. Ways to develop group safety include:

- Establishing and maintaining group norms,
- encouraging conversations about diversity,
- emphasizing confidentiality,
- modeling clear leadership,
- keeping time boundaries and
- employing rapport-building activities.

During the autonomy vs. shame and doubt stage, a child ideally develops a sense of autonomy which allows them to explore their environment. Should this sense of autonomy fail to develop, Erikson theorized the child develops shame and self-doubt for themselves and the world around them (Erikson, 1950). Shame at this stage can create lasting impacts across the lifespan such as the development of internalizing disorders (Muris & Meesters, 2014; Nechita & Szentagotai-Tatar, 2013), dysfunction in school for younger children (Monroe, 2009) and psychological distress in adults with intellectual disabilities (Clapton et al., 2018). Like the basic trust vs. mistrust stage, children presenting for group therapy are at high risk for unsuccessful resolution of this stage. Unsuccessful resolution can lead to lack of initiative, shame for behavior, compulsivity, rigidity and continual doubt of abilities amid new environmental demands. **Addressing shame and doubt during group sessions encourages self-exploration which builds upon psychological safety to help clients explore themselves and the world around them**. Ways to therapeutically work through this stage include:

- self-esteem building activities,
- supportive dyad work between members,
- repeating praise of participatory group behavior,
- supportive group leadership,
- reframing perceived internal failures,
- encouraging strengths which promote internal attributes of success,
- role-playing of skills and
- group brainstorming/problem-solving.

Initiative vs. guilt involves the development of the child's emerging sense of initiative and motivation. Failure to achieve this developmental milestone can result in overwhelming guilt and inhibition that emerges from a sense of low self-worth (Erikson, 1950). Fortunately, self-esteem can be bolstered with therapeutic interventions and impact a child's social functioning, behavior and personality (Haney & Durlak, 1998). Like the two stages before it, children are likely to present with unresolved issues in this area.

Activities which foster a sense of self-worth – like the activities for building autonomy – will help increase initiative, confidence and competence. Self-esteem can be domain-specific and if a child is unable to develop self-esteem in one domain, they may develop it with another such as understanding emotions vs. social skills (Bos et al., 2006). Developing self-worth in any area promotes positive emotional growth. Groups with children, like groups with adults, encourage members to interact with each other and attempt novel social and emotional tasks.

Members who did not successfully resolve this stage may be fearful of trying unfamiliar content and reluctant to attempt group tasks like the honest sharing of feelings. Self-esteem activities can provide a powerful "dose of positivity" which promote autonomy and confidence in children.

Many children enter group treatment for the first time during the stage of Industry vs. inferiority, starting around age six until puberty. Past the very beginning of their cognitive and social growth, at this point in development, the world of children vastly increases with language, socialization, intellectualization and play. During this stage, the primary task of the child is "entrance into life" based on the cultural and societal norms of adulthood (Erikson, 1950, p. 258). During this stage, play represents applied learning of future tasks fundamental for success in a given culture. The vastly changing internal worlds of children can be overwhelming. Building self-confidence for everyday tasks is helpful in this stage to increase a child's overall sense of mastery and industry. During industry vs. inferiority, the following provides confidence to mastery of novel tasks:

- role plays,
- repetitive practice,
- mutual give-and-take helping relationships,
- interactive feedback of tasks and actions,
- social and applied problem-solving of client-specific problems.

Erikson's tasks continue through the lifespan. Modern critiques of Erikson's psychosocial stages challenge the ages and sequential path of stages. Contrary to the stage-wise nature of Erikson's theory, development is not monolithic. While Erikson's stages account for basic tasks during the life span, considerable variability exists within different populations relative to individual, social and cultural aspects. Erikson's theory is seen as male-centric and heteronormative and does not fully encompass the experiences of women and LGBTQIA+ youth (Horst, 1995; Rosario et al., 2006). **We must continue to overlap identity and culture onto development to maximize clinical efficacy in child groups**.

For example, identity development is one of the crucial tasks of puberty into teenage years. Contrary to Erikson's view, numerous paths exist to successful identity development and can begin considerably earlier. Mamie Phipps Clark researched black identity development in young children and found they were aware of their racial identity as early as three years old (Clark & Clark, 1939). Research indicates LGBTQIA+ youth follow multiple formation and integration routes which impact psychosocial adjustment (Rosario et al., 2011). Research across identities is clear that identity integration is related to both social relationships and psychosocial adjustment over time- with direct relevance to long-term identity development starting in childhood.

Revisiting our group, imagine a scenario where the group as a whole is working on positive thinking skills. One concrete way to challenge negative thinking in order to develop a positive sense of self is a concrete activity called *thought flipping*. With this activity, members learn to not accept negative self-talk but explore ways to challenge those thinking patterns and encourage resilience. The group of Jamal, Harry, Hawa, George and Jasmine would require some very basic thought flipping because of their general point in cognitive development. Group members at this age may vary considerably in their understanding of internal dialogue and thought processes. Imagine that the idea of thought flipping was introduced in a previous session. In the example below, all members show an understanding of thought flipping and how to use it as an intervention to help negative thinking patterns. For this session, members were asked to bring in specific thoughts they need flipped around with help from the group.

GROUP LEADER: "Did everybody bring in their thoughts for thought flipping today? (Most of the group nods) For those who didn't, don't worry! We can take a few minutes to write them down. I know this is hard to talk about because some of your thoughts that need to be flipped around may feel sad, angry, or anxious. To start out, I am going to collect all of the thoughts. We are going to practice flipping our thoughts around as a group. That's what we do here in group: we take care of each other!" (Group leader walks over to Jamal)

JAMAL (not wanting to hand in his paper): "Mine's stupid. Just throw it away." (Jamal wads up his paper and throws it on the ground)

JASMINE: "Don't say that! You're my friend!"

GROUP LEADER (picks up wadded paper): "Jamal, I can tell this is very personal. I am going to pick up your paper. Before I look at it, I want you to know that it's okay to feel embarrassed, angry, sad or whatever it is you feel. You have a great friend in Jasmine. Jasmine, it seems like you want to help Jamal feel better. (Jasmine nods) Jamal, would it be okay for our friends in group to help with your thoughts?"

JAMAL (scowling): "I don't care. Aren't you supposed to be in charge here? I thought you were a doctor. More like doctor pathetic."

GROUP LEADER (ignoring insult, reads Jamal's paper): "Ahhhhhh. I see why this is hard to bring up. Friends, we have a really important thought to flip around. I'm going to write it on the board: 'Kids at school don't like me because my skin is black.'"

JIMMY (starts laughing): "Nobody cares about that."

GROUP LEADER (turning to Jimmy, angrily): "Jimmy, it is never okay to laugh at somebody's pain. If I hear you do that again today, I am going to ask you to take a time-out from group and you will not be able to play our game or access the prize box. Do you understand? (Jimmy nods quietly with eyes open wide) Can anybody help flip this thought around?"

JASMINE (raises hand): "I love my black skin! My parents say it's my superpower." (leader writes this on the board)

GROUP LEADER: "That's great! It is one of your many superpowers, Jasmine! Who else can help?"

HAWA (raises hand): "I know! If they don't like my skin, they aren't my friend?"

GROUP LEADER: "Nice, Hawa! How about we add some people who might love you just as you are. Who is that for you, Hawa?"

HAWA: "I love my skin. Is that what you mean?"

GROUP LEADER: "That's a great answer. I might also add our friends in group and family members that love us exactly as we are. (leader writes these on the board) Any others?"

HARRY: "I like you, Jamal! You're my friend!"

GROUP LEADER: "That's very kind of you, Harry. It sounds like you want Jamal to feel good about himself and know that you are there to help. (Harry nods) Okay, Jamal. You have a lot of friends in group who want to help you feel good about yourself and your skin, including me. (Jamal looks up at the group leader) As a White man, I can never understand your experience of being Black. What I can say is your experience is true and valid. Do you understand what I mean by valid? (Jamal nods) I hear that some people in your life do not like you because of the color of your skin and that you feel hurt and angry about it. Is that accurate? (Jamal nods again) Let me summarize what we as a group are saying: Jamal, you are amazing exactly as you are. Your friends here in group and family care about you. Your black skin is a superpower. If people don't like it, they don't deserve to be your friend. (Jamal starts to tear up and runs into a corner of the room to hide, the group leader lets Jamal go and turns to the rest of the group after a moment or two of silence)

Sometimes it is hard for us to love ourselves when other people do not. I want to remind everybody in this group that the color of your skin does not define your worth, your ability, or your entire identity. Do not let others make that definition for you. In group, we never make fun of somebody for how they identify, like the color of their skin. We care about each other and show it. That's why we are practicing thought flipping as a group: to show how we can be good friends and members to our group community. Let's take a quick break so I can talk with Jamal one-to-one.

Social relationships are key to development during childhood and adolescence. This is, in all reality, a significant part of the magical power of group interventions. By creating safe, diverse group environments for children to explore their identities, we facilitate successful identity formation and integration. Group is powerful for children and adolescents solely on the unique, supportive atmosphere. In the example above, group members show mastery of group tasks (thought flipping) and take a community approach to caretaking – something often missed in an individualistic mainstream culture. Part of the value in a social activity such as thought flipping is the intrapersonal learning within individual members and the ways in which members learn social skills indirectly during the activity. Outside of the parameters the leader sets (no making fun of somebody for an identity), the other members now have a basic sense of how to handle talking about issues of identity and how they might feel. This can then be used by individual members in their natural environments should a similar situation arise.

Taking into account Erikson's stages while overlapping identity and culture onto development, it becomes easier to find interventions which target major growth tasks of childhood. Specific interventions for self-worth, competence, initiative, learning novel responses, reciprocal social skills and play help children transcend unresolved areas. Furthermore, interventions such as role plays, repeated practice, rapport-building, maintaining group boundaries and establishing safety are basic group principles which simultaneously address key developmental tasks for children. Just like it was difficult for Jamal to hear positive affirmations about him and his identity, it was vital he received and internalized some portion of them. Think about all of the strategies listed above and how they could create an affirming, open, exploratory space for clients to resolve any 'stuck' points in your groups!

Exercise

1   How did you interpret Jimmy's laughter in response to Jamal's negative thoughts? The clinician above may have missed an opportunity to explore the interaction. Jimmy may have intended it because he doesn't like Jamal and intended to insult him; alternatively, he may have intended to minimize the thought because he likes Jamal and doesn't care about his skin color; Jimmy may feel something similar because of his own skin color. All of these and many more interpretations are possible. Regardless of the interpretation, the clinician missed an opportunity to process and clarify the experience. If you were the clinician, how would you have handled the situation?

2   In what way would you validate Jamal's experiences about people not liking him for the color of his skin within the activity?

3   How else? Would you flip Jamal's thought around in a way he might understand and hear?

4   How does this activity (thought flipping) relate to Erikson's Industry vs. Inferiority stage?

Vygotsky and the Zone of Proximal Development

Compared to most of the previous "classic" theories, Vygotsky heavily emphasized culture. His sociocultural theory suggests individuals learn cultural beliefs and skills through older members in society and is contextually based on culture (Arnett, 2012). He was in many ways a forerunner to modern thinking about development which seeks to conceptualize people using both psychological theory and cultural perspectives. Vygotsky's concept of the "Zone of Proximal

Development" (ZPD) offers a good model for the child group therapist in working with children from a developmental perspective. Similar to the Information Processing Theory which outlines *how* vs. *what* and *when* of cognitive development, the Zone of Proximal Development offers a "how" method of social learning. Group is a uniquely social therapy which hinges on people's innate relational nature. With children, understanding how this is done across childhood and adolescence allows group therapists to better meet the needs of their clients.

The Zone of Proximal Development is defined as "the distance between a child's 'actual developmental level as determined by independent problem-solving' and the higher level of 'potential development' as determined through problem solving under adult guidance or in collaboration with more capable peers" (Vygotsky, 1978, p. 86). This concept offers a method to teach concepts at a developmentally appropriate level. The ZPD has important implications for group therapy with children. **When working with children, there is a constant re-imagining of activities in order to ensure that different members understand therapeutic messages given their individual, unique points in development**.

The movement towards potential development through active support by peers and adults is referred to as *scaffolding* (Berk & Winsler, 1995). Scaffolding is a concept which outlines how an individual who has mastered a task is then directly providing support to somebody learning it. Support can take a lot of different forms. Infants need physical support to learn to walk and may hold their parent's hand until they can walk unassisted. Children learning to write may need to watch their teacher draw the letters before tracing them on their own papers and eventually writing independently. A clinician might practice a relaxation technique with a child who is upset during session to provide an applied example of the skill. All of these examples illustrate how one individual breaks down a concept and helps others understand it. Group leaders with children, just like individual therapists with their clients, can use scaffolding as a tailoring tool for interventions to ensure retention. **Children are capable of showing mastery of advanced relational and intrapersonal skills with appropriate assistance from group leaders**.

Consider the following ways to include scaffolding into your child group practice:

• Strategically pairing members in group activities based on their ability with the specific activity or concept (such as deep breathing)
• Using fish bowls where the group watches several members practice a skill or concept
• Brief psychoeducation "snippets" prior to activities which apply them
• Visual aids
• Anchoring new information to previously learned information
• Reviewing material after learning
• Modeling and/or demonstrating new concepts

A few examples include working on "show and tell" to practice targeted attention with visual aids that say "Attention Here" or "Stop"; comparing and contrasting different emotions "thermometers" where groups identify feelings as they increase in intensity or modeling what it looks like to follow group rules. Because children of similar ages can be at different points of intellectual, social and intrapersonal development, it is critical for child therapists to use skills such as scaffolding to ensure they are understanding content. **Scaffolding encourages clinicians to think about whether children are receiving clinical messages and effectively understanding and applying them**.

Imagine you are the group leader and decide to do a session about the "iceberg analogy." You've seen the group struggle with compound emotions and articulating their experiences into words. Sometimes, you see group members mislabeling emotions in themselves or others without full understanding. Just last session, Jimmy suggested Hawa was feeling bored when she described feeling nervous before a piano recital. You decide the "iceberg analogy" (most of an iceberg is invisible below the surface) will help the group explore multiple emotions and how one emotion can look like another. As you present the idea, it is very obvious the group simply does not understand it. They cannot relate to the iceberg or how certain emotions are "below the surface." In fact, only Jasmine was able to grasp the concept. The rest of the group stopped attending and side conversations increased.

Every clinician has experiences where an intervention, as well planned as it may be, completely flops. In the adult world, these are analogous to misattunement or therapeutic ruptures. Part of working with people is doing your best to create interventions specifically for your client's development. In a scenario such as this one, group leaders have many options. The group is providing feedback that the topic is too advanced. That doesn't mean the content isn't helpful, just above their ability to abstract. Therefore, the issue at hand becomes how to communicate this skill in a way which members can understand.

Thinking on the fly, you choose to reorient and talk about anger masks. Anger is common in the group and co-occurs with multiple other emotions. Using paper plates in your group room, you ask each member to draw what it looks like when they are angry. After showing off their anger masks to the group, you ask them to draw another emotion they feel sometimes, especially before or after they are angry. Jamal drew a sad face which you were able to relate to the last session about thought flipping. Hawa drew a green worried face while saying she gets nervous at school because of bullies. Afterward, you ask them to physically put the anger mask on top of the other emotion and provide some brief psychoeducation about how sometimes people show one emotion but really feel a different one. The group clearly understood this concept and was able to draw several more masks.

Repackaging the content allowed members to successfully identify their own co-occurring emotions. Scaffolding during group takes many forms but always ensures members understand and apply group lessons. By taking feedback during the example above and realizing members were not "getting it," the same idea was reworked in a way which encouraged mastery. While members still required assistance on an individual level, this example represents a group-wide scaffolding to ensure active learning of content.

Imagine the same group is learning about anxiety in order to process, experience, verbalize and better cope with it. Many anxious children show decreased regulation skills which are important to target during treatment (Keil et al., 2017). The group might start by assessing each member's knowledge of anxiety.

GROUP LEADER: "Everybody is doing such a wonderful job talking about their experiences with anxiety. In particular, Hawa, Jasmine and Jimmy showed such great examples and used their listening bodies. Everybody earned two stickers and I am giving an extra one to Hawa, Jasmine and Jimmy. Now that we've talked about what anxiety looks like, it's time to figure out how to help yourself feel better when you're feeling anxious, panicked, nervous or scared. We are going to come up with lists together as partners! I am going to hand out some pieces of paper. Colored pencils and markers will be in the middle of the room, please use one at a time so we share with everybody. I would like each of you to draw or write things you can do to help yourself when you're feeling anxious. Does everybody understand? (the group nods)

"Great. Hawa, you are with George. Jasmine, you are with Jamal. Jimmy, you are with Harry!"

HARRY: "I don't even know what to draw. We are doing what again?"

GROUP LEADER: "Jimmy, do you remember?"

JIMMY: "I'm drawing things I do when I'm anxious."

GROUP LEADER: "That's right. We are writing or drawing ways we can help ourselves feel better when we are anxious."

HARRY: "OH! I think… like when my mom tells me I'm nervous, she puts her hand on my stomach and makes me breath with her. It's SO ANNOYING. Like, stuff like that?"

GROUP LEADER: "Jimmy, what do you think?"

JIMMY (chewing on a marker while he thinks): "Yeah, like that. My mom makes me run laps around the house. OH! And squeeze this super fluffy toy she got me!"

GROUP LEADER: "Great ideas. Come up with as many as you can!"

GEORGE: "I don't feel nervous. I never feel nervous. How can I help myself feel better when I don't feel nervous?"

HAWA (shrugging): "I don't know. You never get scared of storms? I don't know."

GROUP LEADER (walking over to Hawa and George): "It sounds like George is having a tough time thinking about when he has felt any kind of anxiety or fear. Is that right, George?"

GEORGE (nodding): "I just don't get scared."

GROUP LEADER: "Alright. Hawa had a really nice question for you. You've mentioned in group that you don't like storms. Remember when there was a tornado warning during group? You ran and hid under your chair."

GEORGE: "DUH. I didn't want to DIE in a tornado. I wasn't scared."

GROUP LEADER: "What were you feeling?"

GEORGE: "Nothing. I wasn't scared."

HAWA: "You looked scared to me. Your eyes were like this (Hawa exaggerated her eyes to open as wide as possible) and you were shaking."

GROUP LEADER: "I remember that! You also said your hands were sweaty and your heart was beating really fast. That sounds like fear to me. What do you think, Hawa?"

HAWA (nodding in agreement): "George, you were DEFINITELY scared. My hands get all gross when I'm nervous, just like you."

GEORGE: "…"

GROUP LEADER: "Hawa, do you remember how we helped George that day?"

HAWA: "YES. He wanted to be wrapped up like a burrito in one of the blankets. So that's what you did, you made a burrito-George. A George-ito!" (Hawa starts to giggle)

GEORGE (becoming angry): "It's NOT funny!"

GROUP LEADER: "George, I do not believe Hawa is making fun of you. I think she is trying to help. Is that correct, Hawa? (Hawa nods) Alright, it seems like you might be embarrassed by what happened. I want you to know that it is normal to be afraid of storms and tornadoes, and it is always okay to feel. How could you write or draw the idea of wrapping yourself up to feel more comfortable?"

GEORGE (calming down): "I call it blanket time. It always helps me feel better."

HAWA (looking down): "I like blankets, too. They are warm and fuzzy. What color is your blanket at home?"

GEORGE: "It's blue. I need help drawing it."

GROUP LEADER: "Hawa, would you be able to help George after you finish what you're writing down on your list?" (Hawa nods) Thank you! I'm going to check in on Jasmine and Jamal."

JASMINE: "I never thought about that! That's so cool!"

GROUP LEADER: "It looks like you all have quite the list!"

JASMINE: "Yeah! Jamal didn't want to write, but I love writing. I think Jamal was nervous at first. (JAMAL: "I was not!") Now we have like a million things!" (Jamal nods and grins)

GROUP LEADER: "That's so awesome! Tell me a few!"

JASMINE: "Well, Jamal said thought flipping and going outside. I also like to go outside but to play soccer. Jamal plays basketball with his friends or jumps on his trampoline."

GROUP LEADER: "Wow, those are some great ideas! I like that you all are working together so well. We can learn so much from each other when we work together. Jasmine, you talked last week in group about deep breathing. Can you show me and Jamal what that is?"

JASMINE: "Yeah! My mom taught me box breathing. It's like this…"

Within this group, members were strategically placed together based on their comfort with anxiety. At the start of the example, Hawa, Jasmine and Jimmy were identified as members with advanced knowledge of anxiety. They were split up to help scaffold other group members. Vygotsky's principles help clinicians understand how each member is going to respond to group-as-a-whole and individual interventions. In this example, the group leader often relied on scaffolding so that members of the group with advanced emotion recognition were able to help other children in the group. Jimmy helped Harry remember the activity and evaluate some of the coping skills he mentioned; Hawa helped George by pointing out signs of anxiety and coping skills from a previous session and Jasmine helped Jamal by her flexibility with writing and provided a new breathing technique.

Using the Zone of Proximal Development provides opportunities for growth and success. Combining techniques such as scaffolding with healthy group norms encourages a cohesive group. After all, with successful group norms and a safe, brave group space there are high levels of compliance and regulation! Considering a client's current level of competence and cultural values along with realistic possibilities for growth minimizes the chances of 'setting them up for failure.' This also safeguards the therapist's tendency to over-structure therapy groups by allowing for scaffolding work. **Scaffolding can be seen as another form of process work with children since clinicians must pause, evaluate and talk about here-and-now group dynamics**. Oftentimes, group activities take longer than anticipated when attending to how the group as a whole interprets the content. When planning groups, we often repeat the phrase "less is more!" to remind us of the importance of creating time for processing.

When taken together, the power of the group is born from the interconnected learning from peers. The concept of members teaching members leans into the strengths of social learning theories and research. By keeping an eye on a member's zone of proximal development on a given subject, we further comprehend what might be expected in terms of clinical growth. **In this way, we can monitor client outcomes while encouraging evaluation of interventions to ensure they are in service of individual client goals**.

Discussion Questions

1   Think about scaffolding and how you apply it in your groups. How do you practice scaffolding in your child groups?

2   Are there members in your groups who could be helpful as content or emotional leaders on certain topics? How can existing members in your groups act as leaders on specific topics?

3   How does socialization differ within your client's individual families? How does this relate to cultural values and norms within their family?

4   How could you use Bandura's social learning to encourage healthy interpersonal dynamics within your groups?

5   How does social learning relate to group norms?

6   Think about the Zone of Proximal Development. How might you apply this to a group of five-to-seven-year-olds wanting to learn about trauma reactions?

Intrapersonal Development

> It is imperfection - not perfection - that is the end result of the program written into that formidably complex engine that is the human brain, and of the influences exerted upon us by the environment and whoever takes care of us during the long years of our physical, psychological and intellectual development.
>
> Rita Levi-Motalcini, 1988, *In Praise of Imperfection*

As opposed to cognitive and interpersonal development, less consensus exists on the dynamics of intrapersonal personality development and how it relates to targeted areas for interventions such as emotional regulation. Without an overarching theory, clinicians often combine separate ones such as Attachment Theory which detail aspects of intrapersonal development.

Attachment Theory

Attachment Theory, originally developed by John Bowlby, is a bridge between interpersonal and intrapersonal development with implications for both concepts. Attachment Theory proposes that, starting at birth, caregiver sensitivity to the infant's needs impacts social relationships and emotional well-being during childhood and across the life span. Attachment receives considerable research attention, as exemplified by the work of Stern and Beebe (2017) described above, due to the impact of relationships on human development. Broadly speaking, a recent meta-analysis offers important empirical evidence for the notion that secure caregiving in infancy provides greater social competency, fewer externalizing problems (defiance, lying, bullying, delinquency, etc.) and fewer internalizing problems (sadness, anxiety, self-criticism, low self-esteem, etc.) (Groh et al., 2017).

As group therapists, we are often viewed as attachment figures and can thus serve as a consistent, predictable, safe figure during the course of group treatment. Long-term adult-child relationships, like teacher-student, have impacts on attachment including secure exploration of surroundings, socialization and emotional safety (Verscheuren & Koomen, 2012). Leader-member relationships can have a similar impact. Attachment theory considers intimate relationships and their impact on socioemotional development. Therapeutic relationships are intimate, professional relationships which guide clients through challenging experiences. Therapist-client relationships may act as a secure base for clients and, over time, offer benefits of that security. Of course, the professional therapeutic relationship is different from that of parent-child, grandparent-child, aunt-child or even teacher-child. However, the innate healing of healthy relationships is evident across numerous types of therapies and therapeutic relationships (Bell et al., 2016; DeVet et al., 2003; Howgego et al., 2003; Johnson et al., 2005; Mössler et al., 2019; Priebe & McCabe, 2008). The child relationship to the therapist can serve to augment, strengthen or heal insecure attachments that were originally formed at home.

Ainsworth scientifically explored Bowlby's view of attachment by studying infants using the well-known Strange Situation experiment (Ainsworth et al., 1978). Though we know now there are many successful routes to healthy attachments, Ainsworth identified three broad categories (avoidant, secure, ambivalent) of attachment based on how children reacted to the leaving of their parents from the room, interacted with strangers and greeted parents upon their return. A fourth attachment style – disorganized – was subsequently identified by Main and Solomon (1986). The following are broadly considered the predominant theoretical attachment styles:

- **Avoidant attachment**, or those who avoided caregiver interaction and showed little preference for their return;
- **Secure attachment**, or those who showed preference for caregiver and actively sought safety from them;
- **Ambivalent attachment**, or those who showed little preference towards caregivers vs. strangers; and
- **Disorganized attachment**, or those who had little discernible patterns and were difficult to soothe while being largely unpredictable.

Attachment styles often move unimpeded into adulthood. Without intervention, unhealthy attachment styles formed in early life can persist throughout one's lifetime. The overall process of therapy can help insecure attachments to be more secure. Few therapies are better suited to increase secure attachment than group therapy. Most people are securely attached and functionally relate to others. Since attachment impacts one's ability to self-soothe, trust others and form healthy bonds, group relationships become inherently important to group leaders. Healthy group relationships act as a safe, secure base for children, some of whom do not have one outside of the group itself.

Core relational skills such as

- Consistency
- Compassion
- Empathy
- Vulnerability
- Validation
- Active listening

are native skills to therapists and serve to soothe attachment disruptions in child groups. More than anything, this accounts for the relational healing which we know is an integral part of any therapy, especially in groups. ***Healthy relationships are healing***. Understanding attachment, and our client's individual attachment styles, provides an interpersonal road map for individual interventions during group.

Attachment theory is not without notable criticisms which broaden understanding of the ways healthy relationships are formed. Bowlby and Ainsworth's lab-constructed research with white, middle-class mother-infant dyads is limited because they do not encompass the wide range of infant and child-rearing practices around the world which can lead to secure attachment (Vicedo, 2017).

Child-rearing practices vary greatly across cultures and time. For example, co-sleeping is rare in Western child-rearing practices but common for up to 90% of the world; household members vary greatly between different ethnic and cultural groups, even within the same broader city community; make-believe play involves different members of the household based on in-home familial relationships (Berk & Meyers, 2016). Many cultures de-emphasize the immediate attachment between mothers and infants in favor of broader social contexts including extended family and local communities. Paternal affection and involvement is related to positive social and emotional outcomes (Berk & Meyers, 2016) while attachment with extended families and local communities can lead to healthy relational functioning during adulthood. **Attachment, like development, is not monolithic**.

In order to consider how humans develop in relation to one another, we must consider the many paths to achieving healthy social functioning outside of the mother-infant dyad.

Contrary to Ainsworth and Bowlby's work, familiarity and comfort with strangers and larger family or social groups is not pathological, but perfectly normal in certain cultures. This accentuates a key point about relational functioning: **Many routes exist to healthy relational and intrapersonal functioning**. Cross-cultural studies regarding attachment speak to the normalcy of cognitive processes which mediate the adaptation of different relationships as primary, thus evidencing the many routes to a healthy attachment bond with a caregiver (Main, 1990).

Across attachment research, one thing is resoundingly clear: Human contact is important to human development. The exact nature and people involved vary greatly from culture to culture. With our clients, we must understand the cultural contexts they exist within and bring to our groups so we do not perpetuate a narrow view of attachment and relational health.

Exercise

Attachment theory was founded using predominantly white, middle-class samples. How do child-rearing practices differ across cultures? How is attachment different across cultures and how does culture impact views of attachment? How do your individual identities impact your view of attachment?

Think about your own identities and the cultural identities of the following two children. In what ways might you work with their very differing attachment styles while they are in the same group? Describe how you would conceptualize attachment and intervene with each using a relational framework:

Christian is an 11-year-old white, cisgender male from a rural area referred for anger issues. Christian was raised by his grandmother since infancy. His grandfather is deceased and both of his biological parents are unable to provide care (one is in jail and the other is unhoused and struggles with drug addiction). He fights often with his grandmother who becomes frustrated quickly. Other times, he is aloof and distant from her.

Amy is a nine-year-old Chinese-American, cisgender female from a rural area reporting for anger issues. Amy is raised by her biological parents and also lives with her brother, maternal grandparents and uncle. Amy's grandmother often brings her to sessions as her brother has Autism and requires care from her mother and father. Amy's parents are concerned with her anger but are often busy caring for her brother's Autism which severely impairs his day-to-day functioning. Amy appears bonded with her grandmother but is also quick to start arguments with her. Her grandmother becomes frustrated quickly to which Amy typically responds with withdrawing and tears.

Personality Development and Emotional Regulation

Due to its complexity, personality development is enigmatic. While significant literature explores the nature and biological predispositions for personality traits, the processes on the nurture side are murkier. Theorists such as Sidney Blatt (for a synopsis of his prolific research career, see Auerbach, 2017) provide insight into the structure of personality. Blatt suggested a two-factor theory of personality development with relatedness and self-definition as the core dimensions that normally are reciprocally related but that can become exaggerated or distorted in ways that create different kinds of psychopathology and character (Blatt, 2008).

Other trait theories provide biologically based genetic loadings for personality features but do not often account for environmental experiences which change the display of personality traits. For example, Schedler and Westen, the founders of the SWAP-II (Schedler-Westen Assessment Procedure- Second Edition) suggest 14 factors which comprise personality (Westen et al., 2014). However, the complex structures which make up one's personality remain unclear. Without an overarching or clear transtheoretical viewpoint, two basic points remain:

1   **Intrapersonal personality processes relate to emotional regulation, one of the key tasks of childhood; and**
2   **Clinicians must choose how they conceptualize personality and intrapersonal development from their theoretical orientation of choice**.

Group therapists often operate from preferred theories about this aspect of development. For example, psychoanalytic developmental thought includes Blatt's two-factor theory; interpersonal training focuses on the establishment and maturation of needs-focused interaction patterns and cognitive-behavioral theories emphasize the development of schemas and core beliefs which guide thought, feelings and behaviors within one's environment. Each different theoretical orientation offers a unique perspective on personality construction – and is compatible with an interpersonal approach which will be discussed in Chapter 4. All of them provide varying views of personality development which impact or lead to emotional regulation.

Each individual clinician must formulate their own clinical values while identifying a theory from which to operate. Individual theories encourage evidence-based conceptualization such as increasing ego strength, developing complex schemata, or expressing one's needs more appropriately and adaptively. Theories of choice are easily overlapped onto other areas of development to encourage effective regulatory processes.

Across theories, emotional regulation is considered one of the major tasks of childhood. Clinicians may challenge children in group to be successful outside of group by encouraging regulatory processes inside group. By virtue of following healthy group norms, children are also practicing emotional regulation. Being "successful" in group also encourages exploration of the self through feedback from members and leaders. The natural processes within group and ensuing feedback allow for children to learn from each other and develop insight into themselves. In this way, **a variety of approaches may be used to encourage emotional regulation**.

Imagine this interaction from the sample group, where three of your members are working on how to deal with bullies at school:

HARRY: "I have so many bullies at school. Nobody likes me."

JAMAL: "Nobody likes me either. School sucks."

GROUP LEADER: "It sounds frustrating and disheartening to be at school with bullies. I wonder if we can talk as a group about how to handle them so you feel comfortable and confident, even around your bullies. Harry, what is one way you deal with bullies?"

HARRY: "I guess I don't listen to them. But the other day at school we were outside and they were making fun of me for Beyblades."

GROUP LEADER: "That sounds like they were pretty mean. I like that you brought up ignoring them. That's tough to do but an excellent way to handle bullies. When you ignored them, did they go away?"

HARRY: "...yes, after, like, a billion years."

JAMAL: "Honestly though, they stopped. I wish I did that. I always get in trouble because I yell or push them. Sometimes I get so mad that I hit them. They aren't going to hurt me."

GROUP LEADER: "For some people, it is easy to ignore when people are mean. I know I feel sad when people are mean to me. It does get easier with practice, though. I wonder Jamal if you were able to stay calm could you stand up for yourself without yelling or pushing? That way they wouldn't hurt you and you don't get into trouble."

JAMAL (thinking for a moment): "But then they would just hurt me more. Just like when I try to ignore them. They get worse."

GROUP LEADER: "That is a problem. I wonder if the group has any ideas on how to handle this situation?"

GEORGE: "When somebody is mean to me, I tell my teacher. My teachers help me out basically all the time."

GROUP LEADER (nodding): "That's a great idea, George! I think we have stumbled upon a few great techniques which we might be able to try in order. What if we tried ignoring our bullies first, so they don't get a reaction, then speak up for ourselves and ask them to stop, and if they don't tell an adult? Is there a teacher at your school Jamal who you trust?"

JAMAL (thinking for a minute): "Nope. Wait… I like the receptionist, Ms. Allison. She is the nicest person ever."

GROUP LEADER: "That's great! I'm glad you have somebody in your school whom you trust. Harry, what do you think about our three ideas? Could you give them a try at school? It might not fix everything, and it helps to know that you can speak up for yourself."

HARRY (looking down): "I can try I guess."

GROUP LEADER: "I know it's hard to stand up for yourself. I am glad you are willing to try. Can you let us know next week how it goes?" (Harry nods)

Think about what constitutes this concrete, problem-solving activity. Harry is praised for his ability to walk away from frustrating situations. Jamal is actively comparing himself to Harry, noting he has a harder time regulating while confronting bullies. The group leader reinforces both approaches to dealing with bullies, encouraging a softer approach to Jamal while emphasizing emotional regulation. Then, when the problem remains, the group is asked for solutions, with George identifying another interpersonal coping skill for bullies. Hopefully, the members hear that:

a   there are multiple approaches to problems;
b   multiple approaches are not wrong, but vary via situation and person;
c   each person has to take into account their own personality when deciding how they will choose to act in a given scenario; and
d   emotional regulation helps during communication.

Consider your own theoretical orientations and what they say about personality and emotional regulation during development.

Integration of Cognitive, Social and Intrapersonal Development

One thing is clear about working with children: An understanding of human development is no small feat. The lack of defining metatheory for human development creates siloed paradigms which must be inelegantly combined. The vast, ever-expanding body of knowledge of human maturation is simultaneously vital and difficult-to-integrate when styling group interventions. To make it more complex, clinicians must think critically about how development and culture intertwine.

Intersectionality, which will be talked about in greater length in the next chapter, is imperative when integrating various identities and aspects of development. The child therapist must seek to understand an individual's various identities and how their overlap impacts their experiences. A child with an intellectual learning difference will not fall neatly into Piaget's stages but will still actively learn from peers, a child with autism may need additional scaffolding when using modeling as an intervention and a child with ADHD may need additional rehearsal to encode group messages. Even socialization and play are often gendered (Änggård, 2011) – how would socialization and messages about gendered play impact a trans child? Each client is an individual with many identities intersecting in complex ways with their point in development. What is normal for one client is not normal for another.

Clinicians must see, understand and validate overlapping pieces of development and identity. People around the world receive different social and cultural messages which must be honored in the therapy space. As clinicians, we have to use all of our clinical 'lenses' we have to best serve our unique child groups. Integration of the many human development and cultural factors vastly impacts our clinical work and our ability to connect with clients.

Successful child clinicians ask themselves questions which are important to the cross section of development and group interventions:

- *How do I know my interventions are effective?* Are my clients understanding the content of interventions? Are my interventions age-appropriate?
- Am I using too many or too complex explanations and words? Does everybody appear "tuned in?" How can I involve *learning by doing*?
- What are the different identities of my clients and how can I integrate them into my practice? *How does the culture of my clients impact their development?*
- *What are the group norms* for this group? In what ways will I shape or develop healthy group norms?
- *How do I know my group members have a sense of safety and bravery within group?* What interactions led to or, if safety is not established, *not led* to this outcome?
- *Which theory* will be the basis for my group interventions?

Understanding each client facilitates successful group screening, the development of group cohesion and the choosing of meaningful interventions. Continual evaluation of our group interventions, client progress and group dynamics encourages this clinical introspection. As long as we remain open, curious, flexible and educated, we continue to honor our child groups!

Exercise

What would you do? Below are specific scenarios. Imagine yourself as the clinician. How might you respond taking into account all the aspects of development discussed within this chapter?

You have an intake for somebody interested in the sample group used throughout this chapter. They are 11 years old and on the Autism Spectrum. Parents inform you they are 'high-functioning' and have issues with social skills and anger regulation. During the intake, the client is notably more impaired than parents described intellectually, socially and emotionally. They are currently working well below grade-level academics and the client was physically and verbally aggressive during the intake, at one time screaming in the face of a parent and striking their arm for not giving them a toy. How do you handle this scenario? Thinking about the rest of the group, do you allow this client to join your existing group? Why or why not?

Now, imagine you are on your sixth session with this particular group. The group is building a sense of safety. However, this cohesion is still tenuous. As a group, members are working on speaking up for what they need.

HARRY: "I really like superheroes with big muscles. I want to be strong like Iron Man! Can we learn how to do that in group?"

JAMAL: "Iron Man sucks. I hate him. This is dumb. You're dumb, Harry."

HARRY: "You're dumb, Jamal! You and your stupid fire fighters. They don't have any special powers. You're such a loser!"

JAMAL: "Fire fighters are REAL heroes! At least I don't like dumb, STUPID heroes, they aren't even real!"

(Harry throws his pencil at Jamal who gets up and starts to move towards Harry)

In this moment, how would you respond, resolve conflict and encourage positive group norms in a developmentally sensitive way?

Several more sessions later, Hawa decides to quit the group. Her anxiety has markedly decreased and she learned new methods in which to cope. However, another member, Jasmine, is now concerned about being the only girl in the group. How do you handle saying goodbye in a healthy way? How do you manage Jasmine's concern? Who do you feel would be an ideal referral to add to this group and why?

Hopefully, while working through this case example, you see the complexity of development and how it plays out in child groups. Children are not "little adults" as once thought but are capable of incredible feats when provided a brave, nurturing space in which to grow.

References

Ainsworth, M. D. S., Blehar, M. C., Waters, E., & Wall, S. (1978). *Patterns of attachment: A psychological study of the strange situation*. Mahwah, NJ: Lawrence Erlbaum.

Ali, D. (2017). NASPA Policy and Practice Series: Safe Spaces and Brave Spaces, Historical Contexts and Recommendations for Student Affairs Professionals. Retrieved February 26, 2021, from https://www.naspa.org/images/uploads/main/Policy_and_Practice_No_2_Safe_Brave_Spaces.pdf

Änggård, Eva (2011). Children's Gendered and Non-Gendered Play in Natural Spaces. *Children, Youth and Environments*, *21*(2), 5–33. Retrieved from http://www.colorado.edu/journals/cye

Arnett, J. J. (2012). *Human development* (1st ed.). Upper Saddle River, NJ: Pearson Education, Inc.

Ashcraft, M.H. (2009). *Cognition*. Upper Saddle River, NJ: Prentice Hall.

Auerbach, J. S. (2017). The contributions of Sidney J. Blatt: A personal and intellectual biography. *Research in psychotherapy (Milano)*, *20*(1), 222. https://doi.org/10.4081/ripppo.2017.222

Bandura, A. (1965). Influence of models' reinforcement contingencies on the acquisition of imitative responses. *Journal of Personality and Social Psychology*, *1*(6), 589–595. https://doi.org/10.1037/h0022070

Bandura, A. (1977). *Social learning theory*. Englewood Cliffs, NJ: Prentice-Hall.

Bell, H., Hagedorn, W. B., & Robinson, E. H. M. (2016). An exploration of supervisory and therapeutic relationships and client outcomes. *Counselor Education & Supervision*, *55*(3), 182–197. https://doi.org/10.1002/ceas.12044

Bergman, A., Blom, I., Polyak, D., & Mayers, L. (2015). Attachment and separation–individuation: Two ways of looking at the mother–infant relationship. *International Forum of Psychoanalysis*, *24*(1), 16–21. https://doi.org/10.1080/0803706X.2014.893390

Berk, L. E., & Meyers, A. B. (2016). I*nfants, children, and adolescents* (8th ed.). Boston, MA: Pearson Education, Inc.

Berk, L. E., & Winsler, A. (1995). *Scaffolding children's learning: Vygotsky and early childhood education.* Washington, DC: National Association for the Education of Young Children.

Bibace, R. (2013). Challenges in Piaget's legacy. *Integrative Psychological & Behavioral Science, 47*(1), 167–175. https://doi.org/10.1007/s12124-012-9208-9

Bjorklund, D. F. (2018). A metatheory for cognitive development (or "Piaget is Dead" Revisited). *Child Development, 89*(6), 2288–2302. https://doi.org/10.1111/cdev.13019

Blatt, S. J. (2008). *Polarities of experience: Relatedness and self-definition in personality development, psychopathology, and the therapeutic process.* Alexandria, VA: American Psychological Association. https://doi.org/10.1037/11749-000

Bos, A. E. R., Muris, P., Mulkens, S., & Schaalma, H. P. (2006). Changing self-esteem in children and adolescents: A roadmap for future interventions. *Netherlands Journal of Psychology, 62,* 26–33.

Bowlby, J. (1958). The nature of the child's tie to his mother. *International Journal of Psychoanalysis, 39,* 350–371.

Brems, C. (1994). *The child therapist: Personal traits and markers of effectiveness.* Needham Heights, MA: Allyn & Bacon.

Brody, G. (2004). Siblings' direct and indirect contributions to childhood development. *Current Directions in Psychological Science, 13,* 124–126.

Cartwright, K., Galupo, M., Tyree, S., & Jennings, J. (2009). Reliability and validity of the complex postformal thought questionnaire: Assessing adults' cognitive development. *Journal of Adult Development, 16,* 183–189. https://doi.org/10.1007/s10804-009-9055-1

Clapton, N. E., Williams, J., & Jones, R. S. P. (2018). The role of shame in the development and maintenance of psychological distress in adults with intellectual disabilities: A narrative review and synthesis. *Journal of Applied Research in Intellectual Disabilities, 31*(3), 343–359. https://doi.org/10.1111/jar.12424

Clark, K. B., & Clark, M. P. (1939). The development of consciousness of self and the emergence of racial identification in Negro preschool children. *Journal of Social Psychology 10,* 591–599.

Cole, P. M., Tamang, B. L., & Shrestha, S. (2006). Cultural variations in the socialization of young children's anger and shame. *Child Development, 77*(5), 1237–1251. https://doi.org/10.1111/j.1467-8624.2006.00931.x

DeVet, K. A., Kim, Y. J., Charlot-Swilley, D., & Ireys, H. T. (2003). The therapeutic relationship in child therapy: Perspectives of children and mothers. *Journal of Clinical Child & Adolescent Psychology, 32*(2), 277. https://doi.org/10.1207/S15374424JCCP3202_13

Erikson, E. H. (1950). *Childhood and society.* New York: Norton.

Garber, J., Frankel, S. A., & Herrington, C. G. (2016). Developmental demands of cognitive behavioral therapy for depression in children and adolescents: Cognitive, social, and emotional processes. *Annual review of clinical psychology, 12,* 181–216. https://doi.org/10.1146/annurev-clinpsy-032814-112836

González-González, C. S., Gómez Del Río, N., Toledo-Delgado, P. A., & García-Peñalvo, F. J. (2021). Active game-based solutions for the treatment of childhood obesity. *Sensors (Basel, Switzerland), 21*(4). https://doi.org/10.3390/s21041266

Groh, A. M., Fearon, R. M. P., Ijzendoorn, M. H., Bakermans, K. M. J., & Roisman, G. I. (2017). Attachment in the early life course: Meta-analytic evidence for its role in socioemotional development. *Child Development Perspectives, 11*(1), 70–76. https://doi.org/10.1111/cdep.12213

Haney, P. & Durlak, J. A. (1998). Changing self-esteem in children and adolescents: A meta-analytical review. *Journal of Clinical Child Psychology, 27*(4), 423–433, https://doi.org/10.1207/s15374424jccp2704_6

Henrich, J., Heine, S. J., & Norenzayan, A. (2010). The weirdest people in the world? *Behavioral and Brain Sciences, 33,* 61–83.

Horst, E. A. (1995). Reexamining gender issues in Erikson's stages of identity and intimacy. *Journal of Counseling & Development, 73*(3), 271–278. https://doi.org/10.1002/j.1556-6676.1995.tb01748.x

Howgego, I. M., Yellowlees, P., Owen, C., Meldrum, L., & Dark, F. (2003). The therapeutic alliance: The key to effective patient outcome? A descriptive review of the evidence in community mental health case management. *Australian and New Zealand Journal of Psychiatry, 37*(2), 169–183. https://doi.org/10.1046/j.1440-1614.2003.01131.x

Johnson, J. E., Burlingame, G. M., Olsen, J. A., Davies, D. R., & Gleave, R. L. (2005). Group climate, cohesion, alliance, and empathy in group psychotherapy: Multilevel structural equation models. *Journal of Counseling Psychology, 52*(3), 310–321.

Johnson, S. B., Blum, R. W., & Giedd, J. N. (2009). Adolescent maturity and the brain: the promise and pitfalls of neuroscience research in adolescent health policy. *The Journal of Adolescent Health: Official Publication of the Society for Adolescent Medicine, 45*(3), 216–221. https://doi.org/10.1016/j.jadohealth.2009.05.016

Keil, V., Asbrand, J., Tuschen-Caffier, B., & Schmitz, J. (2017). Children with social anxiety and other anxiety disorders show similar deficits in habitual emotional regulation: Evidence for a transdiagnostic phenomenon. *European Child & Adolescent Psychiatry, 26*(7), 749–757. https://doi.org/10.1007/s00787-017-0942-x

Kinney, A. (1991). Cognitive-behavior therapy with children: Developmental reconsiderations. *Rational-Emotive Cognitive-Behavior Therapy 9*, 51–61. https://doi.org/10.1007/BF01060637

Lawless, C. D., McGarry, O., & O'Neill, E. (2019). *What is information Processing theory?* Retrieved February 27, 2021, from https://www.learnupon.com/blog/what-is-information-processing-theory/

Main, M. (1990). Cross-cultural studies of attachment organization: Recent studies, changing methodologies, and the concept of conditional strategies. *Human development, 33*(1), 48–61.

Main, M., & Solomon, J. (1986). Discovery of a new, insecure-disorganized/disoriented attachment pattern. In M. Yogman, & T. B. Brazelton (Eds.), *Affective development in infancy* (pp. 95–124). Norwood, NJ: Ablex.

Miller, G. A. (1956). The magical number seven, plus or minus two: Some limits on our capacity for processing information. *Psychological Review, 63*, 81–97. [Available online from *Classics in the History of Psychology.*]

Miller, P. H. (2011). *Theories of developmental psychology* (5th ed.) New York: W.H. Freeman & Co.

Monroe, A. (2009). Shame solutions: How shame impacts school-aged children and what teachers can do to help. *Educational Forum, 73*(1), 58–66.

Mössler, K., Gold, C., Aßmus, J., Schumacher, K., Calvet, C., Reimer, S., Iversen, G., & Schmid, W. (2019). The therapeutic relationship as predictor of change in music therapy with young children with autism spectrum disorder. *Journal of Autism & Developmental Disorders, 49*(7), 2795–2809. https://doi.org/10.1007/s10803-017-3306-y

Muris, P., & Meesters, C. (2014). Small or big in the eyes of the other: on the developmental psychopathology of self-conscious emotions as shame, guilt, and pride. *Clinical Child & Family Psychology Review, 17*(1), 19–40. https://doi.org/10.1007/s10567-013-0137-z

Nechita, D., & Szentagotai-Tatar, A. (2013). Shame and psychopathology: From research to clinical practice. *Journal of Cognitive and Behavioral Psychotherapies, 13,* 101.

Okur, Z. E., & Corapci, F. (2016). Turkish Children's Expression of Negative Emotions: Intracultural Variations Related to Socioeconomic Status. *Infant & Child Development, 25*(5), 440–458. https://doi.org/10.1002/icd.1945

Oles, T. (1991). Matching therapeutic style with developmental level: A guide for child care workers. *Journal of Child and Youth Care, 6*(3), 63–72.

Önder, M. (2018). Contribution of plays and toys to children's value education. *Asian Journal of Education and Training, 4*(2), 146–149.

Perrier, F. (2004). Practising active science with child refugees: A clinical perspective. The *Science Education Review, 3*(2), 67–87.

Piaget, J., & Inhelder, B. (1969). *The psychology of the child*. New York: Basic Books.

Priebe, S., & Mccabe, R. (2008). Therapeutic relationships in psychiatry: The basis of therapy or therapy in itself? *International Review of Psychiatry, 20*(6), 521–526. https://doi.org/10.1080/09540260802565257.

Prinstein, M. J., Youngstrom, E. A., Mash, E. A., & Barkley, R. A. (2019). *Treatment of disorders in childhood and adolescence* (4th ed.). New York: The Guilford Press.

Riester, A. E., & Kraft, I. A. (Eds.). (1986). *Child group psychotherapy: Future tense.* Madison, CT: International Universities Press.

Rodriguez Buritica, J. M., Eppinger, B., Schuck, N. W., Heekeren, H. R., & Li, S.-C. (2016). Electrophysiological correlates of observational learning in children. *Developmental Science, 19*(5), 699–709.

Rosario, M., Schrimshaw, E. W., Hunter, J., & Braun, L. (2006). Sexual identity development among gay, lesbian, and bisexual youths: consistency and change over time. *Journal of Sex Research*, *43*(1), 46–58. https://doi.org/10.1080/00224490609552298.

Rosario, M, Schrimshaw, E. W., Hunter, J. (2011). Different patterns of sexual identity development over time: implications for the psychological adjustment of lesbian, gay, and bisexual youths. *The Journal of Sex Research*, *48*(1), 3–15. https://doi.org/10.1080/00224490903331067.

Scott-Janda, E., & Karakok, G. (2016). Revisiting piaget: Could postformal thinking be the next step? *Philosophy of Mathematics Education Journal*, *30*, 1–11.

Shonkoff, J. P., & Phillips, D. A. (Eds.). (2000). *From neurons to neighborhoods: The science of early childhood development*. Washington, DC: National Academy Press.

Sowell, E. R., Thompson, P. M., Holmes, C. J., Jernigan, T. L., & Toga, A. W. (1999). In vivo evidence for post-adolescent brain maturation in frontal and striatal regions. *Nature neuroscience*, *2*(10), 859–861. https://doi.org/10.1038/13154

Stern, D. N. (1971). A microanalysis of mother-infant interaction. *Journal of the American Academy of Child and Adolescent Psychiatry*, *10*, 501–517.

Swanson, D. P., Spencer, M. B., Harpalani, V., Dupree, D., Noll, E., Ginzburg, S., & Seaton, G. (2003). *Psychosocial Development in Racially and Ethnically Diverse Youth: Conceptual and Methodological Challenges in the 21st Century*. Retrieved from http://repository.upenn.edu/gse_pubs/2

Verschueren, K., & Koomen, H. M. Y. (2012). Teacher–child relationships from an attachment perspective. *Attachment & Human Development*, *14*(3), 205–211. https://doi.org/10.1080/14616734.2012.672260

Vicedo, M. (2017). Putting attachment in its place: Disciplinary and cultural contexts. *European Journal of Developmental Psychology*, *14*(6), 684–699. https://doi.org/10.1080/17405629.2017.1289838

Vygotsky, L. S. (1978). *Mind in society*. Cambridge, MA: Harvard University Press.

Vygotsky, L. S. (1987). The genesis of higher mental functions. In R. Reiber (Ed.), *The history of the development of higher mental functions* (Vol. 4, pp. 97–120). New York: Plenum.

Westen, D., Waller, N. G., Shedler, J., & Blagov, P. S. (2014). Dimensions of personality and personality pathology: Factor structure of the Shedler-Westen Assessment Procedure-II (SWAP-II). *Journal of Personality Disorders*, *28*(2), 281–318. https://doi.org/10.1521/pedi_2012_26_059

Yalom I. D., & Leszcz M. (2020). *The theory and practice of group psychotherapy* (6th ed.). New York: Basic Books.

Zmyj, N., & Seehagen, S. (2013). The role of a model's age for young children's imitation: A research review. *Infant & Child Development*, *22*(6), 622–641. https://doi.org/10.1002/icd.1811

3 Multiculturalism for Child Group Therapy

Zachary J. Thieneman

Introduction

Culture is often considered the "air we breathe" or the "water in which we swim." It is inexorably linked to our understanding of ourselves, our values, our actions and even our perceptions. Culture is deeply ingrained into our experience and impacts communication, relationships, individualism vs. communalism, beliefs, roles, understanding of pathology and every aspect of the human experience. What may not be readily apparent is the way in which cultures differentiate from each other and how an individual develops over time within their culture. This is especially true with **children who receive cultural messages that are normal to them and are not universal to others**. Culture is woven into every fiber of children's beings and the messages they internalize start during infancy, stemming from their immediate environments.

This chapter covers several broad areas for multiculturalism in child groups:

- **Models for cultural conceptualizations, unpacking client and clinician identities and intersecting identities** (Historical biases in behavioral science, Layered Ecological Model, ADDRESSING model, Cultural Humility)
- **Identity development in childhood** (models for identity development; parent-child environment, cultural socialization)
- **How to talk about diversity in child groups including microaggression, power and privilege** (creating brave spaces, handling microaggressions, microaffirmations)
- **The importance of language during child groups** (staying up-to-date with language, glossary of terms)

As discussed during the development chapter, an understanding of where any child is in the group and what interventions would be effective require an assessment both of the developmental stage and appreciation of cultural influences. **Children operate from an egocentric worldview, meaning they believe their "normal" experiences are universal to others, including cultural norms** (a.k.a. the "air" they breathe). This chapter seeks to explore cross-cultural formulations, identity development in children and dynamics of power and privilege which are found in any group – and how to address them in your child groups. While reading this chapter, consider the various differences in your clients, how dynamics of privilege and power play out in your groups, and how you can plant seeds of positive identity development which can grow throughout adolescence and into adulthood. Also, consider *your* demographics and how the richly layered and beautiful components of you affect how you see the world, interact with others, and choose theories and interventions for your clients.

DOI: 10.4324/9781003189701-3

Historical Biases

A family's culture necessarily entails taking a generational perspective. Present-day contexts are directly related to an individual or family's unique cultural history. Looking through the lens of history provides vital information about dynamics of power, privilege and culture.

Psychotherapy is steeped in majority culture stemming from White/European, neurotypical, heteronormative, Christian, gender binary, individualistic, patriarchal traditions. **Acknowledging contextual, historical privilege is an important first step** for our groups in a world of unacknowledged Western privilege. In order to best serve diverse populations, especially children, **acknowledgment and identification of privilege and how it plays out today is a requisite skill**. After this acknowledgment, clinicians must work to make behavioral science more equitable by actively advocating for clients, dismantling systems of oppression in which therapists operate and applying knowledge of client culture to therapy.

Fundamental research in human behavior fields based on WEIRD populations (Western, educated, industrialized, rich and democratic; Henrich, 2010) begs the question: What parts of the human experience are universal and which ones are innately tied to identity and culture? Originally, cultural competence sought to answer that question as it became readily apparent the WEIRD population is a small sliver of human experience. Cultural competence emphasized knowing as much as possible about a given population, creating an initial assumption that proficiency can be acquired through learning all there is to know, while respecting diverse cultures. However, the sheer volume and rapid shifts of cultural environments in addition to individual variations amongst members within a particular demographic make it impossible to attain true and absolute cultural competence. Making assumptions about an individual within a certain identity or culture can be dangerous and create therapeutic ruptures such as microaggressions, thus the idea of cultural competence is now seen as outdated.

Conceptual shifts lead to the idea of cultural humility, or an emphasis on what people don't know about a client rather than making blanket assumptions about a given culture, often from a clinician's culture of origin. Some aspects of humanity are universal, while others are not. Individuals need to be seen as the changing, fluid humans they are. **Applying this concept to group therapy, we must also ask about the universality of interventions and whether culture-specific adaptions must be made, just as we would with individual clients**.

Discrimination is widely apparent in every aspect of culture. Available research paints a bleak picture of the impact of discrimination and prejudice across all areas of identity. For example, black children reporting racial discrimination experience accelerated aging and are at higher risk for depression in young adulthood (Carter et al., 2019). People with intellectual disabilities are often desexualized and not allowed to explore their own sexuality (Sommarö et al., 2020). Many American children's books about Islam show Muslim individuals as monolithic others (Torres, 2016). Transgender youth experience high rates of minority stress and co-occurring internalizing disorders (Turban & Ehrensaft, 2018).

However, research continues to blossom relative to dynamics of power and the reciprocal relationship between individual and culture. Identity research illuminates how understanding people's specific experiences actually expands best practices in working with diverse clients (American Psychological Association, 2017). Several examples illustrate this point. In the past ten years, research on gender identity and expression has increased dramatically (Turban & Ehrensaft, 2018) as have standards of care for gender diversity. Learning about racism and white privilege during structured courses can motivate identity development and orientation to action (Kernahan & Davis, 2010). Better understanding of the dynamics of power and privilege is also a call to better serve diverse clients. **Group leaders are uniquely positioned to positively impact child groups through recognizing and honoring cultural development in children**.

A history of prejudice must be acknowledged to move forward. Acknowledging history creates visibility for the oppression of harmful "isms" which led to generations of trauma and impacts present-day clients. Mental health clinicians are tasked with learning about and from the past to better help clients heal into the present and future.

Starting Points for Multiculturalism

The American Psychological Association has released several iterations of multicultural guidelines similar to other human services organizations including the American Counseling Association's (ACA) *Multicultural and Social Justice Counseling Competencies: Guidelines for the Counseling Profession* (Ratts et al., 2016) and the National Association of Social Worker's (NASW) *Standards and Indicators for Cultural Competence in Social Work Practice* (National Association of Social Workers, 2015). Each of these standards provides valuable education about working with diverse populations and bring culture-focused evidence-based practice to the forefront of psychotherapy.

Defining culture is no easy task given the complexity and intersectionality of identities. No universal definition exists which encompasses the numerous dimensions of culture. APA (2003) offers a list of many such dimensions among peoples:

- Race
- Ethnicity
- Language
- Sexual Orientation
- Gender
- Age
- Disability (now referred to as 'ability differences')
- Socioeconomic Status
- Education
- Religious Orientation/Spirituality

Children, based on their identity and developmental level, assume their experiences are universal. A child who likes weather patterns may assume everybody else does and find it odd if peers don't have a "favorite weather." A child growing up with lesbian parents may assume all children grow up with two mothers because it is their individual experience. Children's egocentric assumptions add a delicate, complex layer when discussing identities during group sessions. Furthermore, **each group member enters with their own set of values, beliefs and experiences which may differ from those of the clinician and other group members with the same identity**. Just like we cannot assume we know the experiences of others different from ourselves, **we cannot assume two children with the same identity have the same experiences**. Two children with Down Syndrome may have completely separate experiences of discrimination, prejudice and exclusion in their environments.

Group clinicians from dominant and non-dominant cultures alike must learn to find opportunities to explore differences to facilitate client growth. Children are no exception and, just as they may be surprisingly intelligent and relational, can be acutely aware of diversity. For group psychotherapy to truly be a universal intervention, we must constantly seek new ways to reach our diverse clients and help the group explore inter-member differences, starting with children.

Layered Ecological Model of the Multicultural Guidelines

The *Multicultural Guidelines: An Ecological Approach to Context, Identity, and Intersectionality* (APA, 2017), published by the American Psychological Association by Clauss-Ehlers et al. (2019), offers a helpful conceptual framework for broad psychological practice (consultation, treatment, research, etc.) called the Layered Ecological model of Multicultural Guidelines. This model is a helpful complement to treatment which encourages clinicians to think systemically. Influenced by Bronfenbrenner's ecological systems theory (1979), the guidelines propose a dynamic, relational movement between the clinician and client centered around the self-definition of both client and clinician. Bronfenbrenner's ecological systems theory is comprised of five concentric circles:

- **Microsystem**: The immediate, bidirectional surroundings of a child such as parents, caregivers, teachers, peers, siblings, etc.
- **Mesosystem**: Interrelations between social relationships in the microsystem, such as caregivers talking with teachers.
- **Exosystem**: Societal and other cultural structures which contain but are not directly influencing a child such as media, neighborhoods, parental workplaces, etc.
- **Macrosystem**: A child's overall cultural context including values, beliefs, and norms also seen in the child's identities.
- **Chronosystem**: Historical context, trends and transitions which impact a child's life over time.

The Layered Ecological Model of the Multicultural Guidelines encourages clinicians to think about the complex systems in each child's life and how they interact with their identities including five layers: Bidirectional Model of Self-Definition and Relationships; Community, School, and Family Contexts; Institutional Impact on Engagement; Domestic and International Climate; and Outcomes. This model emphasizes intersectionality and the complex, bidirectional nature of systems. All of the layers reference the bidirectional impact of systems within which a client exists including the bidirectional relationship between clinician and client. Child clinicians are often accustomed to thinking *systemically*, or using the broader social and cultural factors at large within a child's life, to conceptualize and intervene. The Layered Ecological Model provides a framework for relevant systems and multicultural layers worth considering when working with child groups. Think about the following examples:

Microsystem: Children's relationship(s) with their primary caregivers has important implications for their social functioning. How might a child's relationship with their caregivers impact their presentation during group? In what ways could a child's relationship with their primary caregiver have an effect on the ways they interact with group leader(s)? What about with other group members?

Mesosystem: How would a teacher talking to a caregiver impact a child client? How would a consultation with a teacher specifying helpful interventions impact the child at school and their presentation in group sessions?

Exosystem: The media can vastly impact people's perceptions. How could mass media following a terrorist attack negatively impact a child of North African, Middle Eastern or Eastern European descent who has brown skin?

Macrosystem: In what ways does the public education system impact children differently based on their socioeconomic status?

Chronosystem: In what ways would specific events, such as a child at age 9 leaving his familiar home and neighborhood and moving to another part of the country, impact their mental health?

Children receive messages about themselves and their identities *constantly*. Movies, video games, television, news, social media, music, local governments, international politics, family dynamics and schools all impact children's sense of self. To think systemically is to identify the sources and content of those messages and how they directly affect group dynamics, client presentations and group interventions. A child presenting with anxiety might constantly watch the news and fear global conflict; another child may feel sadness about human rights violations in their country; a third child may not want to self-identify on the LGBTQIA+ spectrum because of pop music they hear on the radio or anti-LGBTQIA+ family messages; or a child in group may shut down when somebody makes a joke about them because they are bullied at school. These examples show the power of systemic influences on child clients who have to navigate cultural messages, often without realizing their influence, all the time. The Layered Ecological Model provides the child clinician with a multicultural framework of systems to attend to including the broader social/cultural climate and community/school/family. These systems vastly affect clients and their presentation. In attending to these systems, both within the group and outside of the group child therapists have the power to intervene more effectively. The Layered Ecological Model includes three processes which detail the interchange between various systems:

- **Power/privilege**: Social power dynamics and privilege experiences by both the clinician and client and within the therapeutic relationship;
- **Tension**: Tensions amongst the different relationships and intersections in the client's life not unique to the therapeutic relationship but pertaining to any or all interactions between systems in the client's life. For example, tension or discord between a child's self-identities and the cultural identity of their family, such as an LGBTQIA+ child in a disapproving religious family;
- **Fluidity**: Changes and shifts between the different concentric circles. An example is the passage of time. Over the course of therapy, children may learn to interact differently with some of the systems in their life and deal with tension more effectively (Figure 3.1).

The Layered Ecological Model is a comprehensive guideline which encompasses aspects of identities and layers of culture relevant to child clients. **As part of a client's**

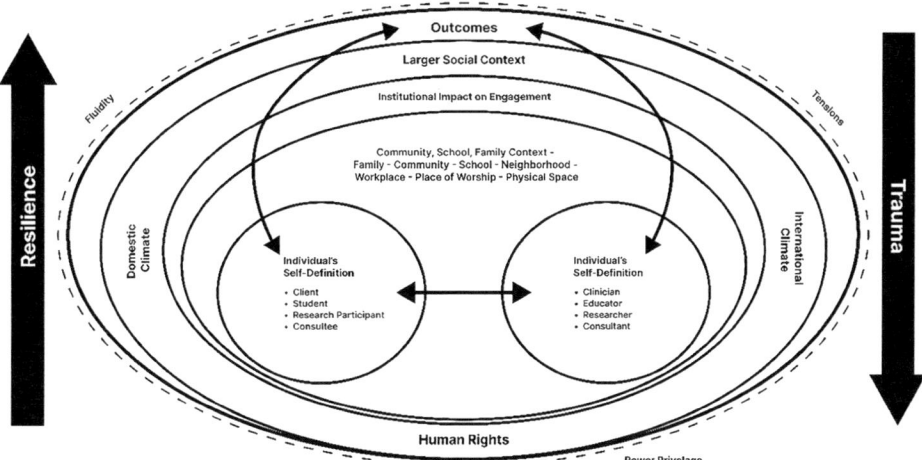

Figure 3.1 Layered Ecological Model of the Multicultural Guideline

microsystem or mesosystem, we have an impact on their well-being and must take into account the various cultural messages they are receiving in their natural, community and societal environments. The child therapist is tasked with cognizance and respect of multicultural variables which dynamically impact children and their presentation.

Exercise

Cultural formulation: Think about a child client with whom you work. Write down their initials on a sheet of paper. Moving outward, make concentric circles for each of the microsystem, mesosystem, exosystem, macrosystem, and chronosystem. Using what you know about the client, fill in each circle with the various cultural contexts for your client. After you are finished, write down a brief cultural conceptualization of the client as a whole which addresses the various systems the client exists within and how they impact the client's presentation. Does this conceptualization change the way you think about the client's pathology or symptom presentation, or your choices of interventions? Why or why not?

Understanding Our Biases Using the Addressing Model

Hays' ADDRESSING model (2001) is a framework to actively identify and discuss dynamics of privilege and power within and between clinicians and clients. **ADDRESSING (Age, Development Disabilities** (please note that as of writing the most current language is 'developmental differences')**/Disabilities acquired, Religion/spirituality, Ethnic/racial identity, Socioeconomic status, Sexual orientation, Indigenous heritage, National origin, Gender)** provides a clear map for identity exploration by outlining common identities and their relation to power and privilege (Figure 3.2).

A Note on Intersectionality

The ADDRESSING model showcases overlapping identities considered with the term *intersectionality*. **Intersectionality, coined by Kimberlé Crenshaw in 1989, identifies the framework for how an individual's overlapping identities variably affect experiences of discrimination and privileg**e. For example, women in academic leadership may face gender-based discrimination while women of color in the same role may face gender and race-based discrimination (Chung et al., 2018). Intersectionality encourages clinicians to think of clients as multidimensional cultural beings with layers of identities and preferences which interact in unique ways. Intersectionality vastly impacts people's experiences. Women of color have vastly different experiences than white women in relation to physical, sexual, and structural violence (Crenshaw & Bonis, 2005). This has important implications for group dynamics. It is critical for therapists to consider the nature of intersecting identities child clients bring to group dynamics.

ADDRESSING Model and Client Identity

Hays' model provides a concrete framework for children to examine their identities. ADDRESSING can help child clients articulate their experiences with power and privilege. Child

Cultural Characteristic	More Power	Less power
Age and Generational Influences	Adults	Children, adolescents, elders
Disability at birth (may have impacted development)	Able-bodied, cognitive functioning intact, no sensory impairments, healthy	Individuals with limitations or disabilities, psychiatric conditions
Disability, acquired after birth and later in life	Able-bodied, cognitive and sensory functioning intact	Purpose, budding initiative
Religion	Christian or Secular	Muslim, Jewish, Hindu, Buddhists,Indigenous, and other minority religions
Ethnic and Racial Identity	Euro-American	People of Color (Asian, Latino, African, African-American, Middle Eastern, Indigenous, other non-white or European ethnicity)
Socioeconomic status	Upper Class & Middle Class (professional, educated, safe living environment with access to and ability to pay for essentials and services)	Poor & Working Class (occupations, access to accurate information, rural or inner city).
Sexual Orientation	Heterosexuals	Gay, Lesbians, Bisexuals, Transgendered, Asexual Individuals
Indigenous Heritage	Non-native	Native
Native (or national) Origin	U.S. born	Immigrants & Refugees
Gender	Men	Women, Queer, Transgendered, Intersex, other non-male identities

Figure 3.2 ADDRESSING: A Model of Cultural Influences and their Relationship to the Social Construct of Power

clients cannot typically describe experiences of privilege and disadvantage in the abstract way adults can, but children experience them nonetheless. For example, children on the autism spectrum may have clear experiences outside of group where they are excluded or bullied for being autistic. **Concrete examples such as identity-related bullying can be extrapolated as examples of power and privilege**. Connecting individual experiences to abstract concepts facilitates identity development in children.

Connecting concrete experiences to abstract ideas promotes understanding of complex concepts. With children, validating these experiences nourishes positive self-identity and provides opportunities to repair harmful impacts of "isms." For the autistic child who is bullied, simply talking about the experience validates and challenges the impact it can have. In a cohesive group, other group members may contest bullying behavior while encouraging a positive autistic identity. Simple statements from other group members such as "That kid stinks. You are the best just as you are!" hold a surprisingly powerful, reparative effect. **Part of the power in child groups is the ability to counteract negative experiences outside of the group by authentic validation of clients, just as they are**.

Unpacking Clinician Identity and Bias

The ADDRESSING acronym implicates the importance of both clinician and client identities. Therapists must unpack their own biases to see stereotypes, "othering," and microaggressions within their groups. Just as therapists clinically consider the impact of identity on client experiences, they must equally weigh their own privileges and how it impacts their personal and professional lives.

Everybody has biases. Bias is deeply ingrained and indoctrinated from a young age until it becomes virtually invisible. The "air we breathe" can be toxic. In his book *Stamped from the Beginning: The Definitive History of Racist Ideas in America*, Ibram X. Kendi (2016) uses the history of racism in America to identify how racial discrimination leads to racist ideas which then leads to ignorance and hate. In other words, systems of oppression create racist attitudes which are promulgated throughout mainstream culture. **As a starting point, clinicians must develop awareness and accept areas of privilege and marginalization**. When we become aware of those biases, we can understand how they play out in our lives and the interactions with our clients.

Caregivers and guardians are frequently the first line of communication with child clients. As any child clinician will report, interactions with caregivers can be exceptionally challenging. If therapists unpack their countertransference reactions to caregivers, they might see their own biases about how caregivers "should" interact with children.

While this may be layered in how the clinician was parented or how they choose to parent their own child, caregiver countertransference often entails feelings, especially negative and critical evaluations, about the child-rearing of their clients. Therapists must remain observant of their own biases so as not to overly pathologize culturally relevant behavior including parenting practices. **We cannot escape our biases, but we can work to understand them and how they impact our client work**. Without a true exploration of identities, it is easy for individuals with privilege to fear conversations surrounding that privilege in a defensive manner exemplified in concepts such as *white fragility* (DiAngelo, 2011).

A non-defensive, honest, open exploration of privilege facilitates a deeper understanding of the self and the historical contexts which have created successes and barriers, personally and professionally. Hays (2016) recommends clinicians explore their own identities to better accept and understand client experiences.

Exercise

Take a moment and write the word ADDRESSING vertically descending on a sheet of paper. Write down your own identities relative to Hays' model. How do you identify in terms of areas of privilege and disadvantage? How have/how do areas of privilege and disadvantage impact your personal and professional worlds? How does understanding your own areas of power impact your ability to see client experiences?

Cultural Humility: Reframing the Conversation

Cultural humility is a modern concept applied as a culturally sensitive communication framework. For example, the National Child Welfare Workforce Institute (www.ncwwi.org) encourages cultural humility in all areas of child welfare. Originally discussed in contrast to cultural competence, **cultural humility was initially created by Melanie Tervalon and Jann Murray-García** in 1998 for physicians working with diverse populations. Since then, the idea of cultural humility has expanded exponentially. Cultural humility is a part of a **multicultural orientation framework** (Hook et al., 2017) which includes three major points:

- **Cultural humility**: seeking and understanding an accurate perception of clinician's individual cultural values and a respectful, attuned, other-oriented therapeutic perspective.
- **Cultural opportunities**: chances in therapy to explore identity and cultural beliefs.
- **Cultural comfort**: feelings before, during and after culture-focused therapist-client conversations.

Reframing the conversation from knowing everything we can about every culture to seeing our limitations of not knowing allows us to see our clients as individuals. Cultural humility encourages us to curiously and openly learn about our clients in relation to their cultures without assumption. Cultural humility is linked to client outcomes including treatment efficacy and working alliance (Davis et al., 2016). Culturally humble therapists do the following (Hook et al., 2017):

- **Identify and continually introspect** on their own values, biases and assumptions;
- Reflect/consider how their **values interact with clinical decisions**;
- Are **open to feedback** from others, including clients;
- Express openness and **curiosity about other's cultural values**;
- **Abstain from presumptions** about the experiences or beliefs of others based on one identity.

Cultural humility includes three major factors (Waters & Asbill, 2013):

- A lifelong commitment to cultural self-exploration, self-evaluation, and self-critique;
- The desire to fix power imbalances;
- Aspiring to partner and develop relationships with advocates (individuals, groups, organizations) who are striving for social equity.

Taken together, the focus of cultural humility is stripping away what we think we know about cultural variations and becoming comfortable with what we don't know. Given our own unique experiences, we cannot pretend to know somebody else's. What we don't know is exactly what we must be open to learning- directly from our clients. As clinicians, even more so with children, we are advocates ensuring they are seen, heard, validated and valued. Operating from a cultural humility standpoint, clients are seen for their unique identities and experiences.

   Cultural humility is vital to child groups. Oftentimes, clinicians view children as too young to adequately process and identify values of their own. However, as discussed in the previous chapter on development, children are dynamic, relational beings with unique identities of their own closely tied to their cultural upbringing. **Children view their environment, whatever that may be, as normal to them and universal to others**.

   The impact of nurture is strong. Children often communicate similarly to their parents (Fivush & Wang, 2005). As a result, children struggle to see different perspectives and routines which aren't part of their immediate day-to-day environments. A stance of cultural humility in child groups often takes the form of scaffolded perspective-taking, group process and content focused on diversity in order to help clients see diverse perspectives and ways of being which gently challenge their inherent worldviews.

The celebration of holidays is a wonderful example illustrating cultural humility in child groups. Holidays enable perspective-taking and cultural identity development with children because they are concrete, specific, annual traditions. Younger children are better able to grasp the concrete, repeated nature of holidays as compared to the belief systems which holidays honor (in contrast to holidays, belief systems are highly abstract). Holidays therefore represent cultural opportunities in child groups!

In a Christian-dominated North American society, holidays such as Christmas are commonly observed. For Christian group members, discussing the meaning of this holiday is an important exercise. Even more important is recognizing and valuing the religious practices of everybody else in the group to ensure other religious identities are seen and valued. As group leaders with children, **modeling openness and curiosity sets a powerful example**.

Jewish members may attend a group session during, before or after Hanukkah. Children talking about their experiences with Hanukkah and family-specific traditions they have surrounding the holiday is a cultural opportunity to explore difference and diversity. Non-Jewish members learn about Hanukkah which can deepen member-to-member relationships and promote a safe space for the group to express the diversity of religious identities in the group- all from facilitating a discussion about a holiday. Throughout the year, holidays present plenty of cultural opportunities. At the end of the year alone, Kwanzaa, Christmas, Hanukkah, Bodhi Day, Pancha Ganapati, Winter Solstice and others all occur within weeks of each other! **Allowing space to recognize and celebrate diversity within a group builds cohesion and visibility**.

> ### Exercise
>
> The following is a vignette of a cultural opportunity revolving around Rami, an 11-year-old Egyptian-American Muslim child celebrating Ramadan in a majority Christian child group.

Picture yourself as Rami. In many areas of your life such as school, people do not appear to understand or care about your Muslim identity which is very important to you and your family. Some teachers are kind, respectful and curious. Most days at best, people don't pay attention to your Muslim identity or ask questions about it, even during your afternoon prayer when you leave class for wudhu (ritual body-washing just before prayer). At worst, people mock you for the clothes you wear, the food you eat, your prayers or your religious celebrations. More than once, kids laughed at you for not celebrating Christmas. You feel like your therapy group sees and is curious about your religion. You feel bonded to the other members and leaders. Before reading this vignette, take a moment to immerse yourself in Rami's perspective. Think about Rami's daily experiences surrounding Islam and what they are like. The following interaction takes place in a group session towards the end of Ramadan.

GROUP LEADER 1: "Rami, your parents told us you are currently celebrating Ramadan. I think the group would like to learn about Ramadan since one of the unique things about you is that you're the only person in here who is Muslim. We love that about you and want to hear about important parts of your life! Can you tell us about Ramadan and how you celebrate?"

RAMI (looking nervous): "…okay. Ramadan is special. We don't eat during the day. My dad says it's to purify our bodies and be strong. I still eat a little sometimes, but only like a snack if I'm REALLY hungry or some water after gym class. It's special and hard at the same time."

GROUP LEADER 2: "Thanks for sharing! Tell us more about fasting. When are you able to eat?"

RAMI: "We eat before the sun comes up and after the sun goes down. It's a LONG time. I eat early in the morning and I eat at night when it's dark out."

CHRIS: "So, you don't eat lunch or anything? How do you even do school?"

RAMI: "I get tired a lot. But the school lets me take breaks and if I get too tired I just eat a snack. Only adults HAVE to fast from when the sun is up until sunset. Except for my mom, she's pregnant. She can eat because she needs to feed both her AND the baby. If anybody is sick or anything, they don't have to fast, either."

CHRIS: "Why do you fast again? And when does Rama-dama-thing end?"

GROUP LEADER 2: "Ramadan, Chris. Please be respectful!"

CHRIS: "Sorry, Ramadan."

RAMI: "My dad says it's to 'cleanse the soul.' I don't know what that means, but it's something to do with being strong to resist the things which may make us bad on the inside. And it's so LONG. Ramadan is a whole MONTH and it changes time every year, I think."

GROUP LEADER 1: "Yes, your mom says it moves up a few weeks each year. Right now it's in the winter, and in a few years, it will be in the fall. That's so cool! Does anybody have any questions?"

CHRIS: "Wait a second. It's dark out now! Can we eat during group?"

GROUP LEADER 2: "That's a great idea. It's called an Iftar, right? The food you eat at night during Ramadan when you break your fast?"

RAMI (eyes lighting up): "Yeah! It's the Iftar! It's basically the best meal ever."

GROUP LEADER: "We might not be able to have an Iftar quite like you do at home or with your mosque community, but it sounds like the group wants to celebrate with you. Is that accurate, group? (group members nod) Maybe we can have some snacks next week and you can take some leftovers to your family? Would that be okay?"

RAMI: "YES! I LOVE chocolate, it's my mom's favorite too. Can we have chocolate?"

GROUP LEADER 1: "We can have chocolate! We will also have a few other snacks since some of our friends don't eat chocolate or have food allergies. I'll talk to you and your mom after group is done and we can figure out the rest of the details. I am glad we can celebrate with you!"

Continue to keep yourself in Rami's shoes. How did you feel about how the group leader brought up Ramadan? Were you comfortable sharing your experiences? What could the group do to help you feel more comfortable talking about your Muslim identity? How did it feel for your group peers (in this case Chris) to take in interest in your Muslim identity? Conversely, how would it feel if they actively did not? What feeling came up when the group leaders offered to bring in food for consumption during your next group meeting's Iftar?

Identity Development in Children

Children's social and intellectual abilities are often underestimated given the fluid nature of development and variation amongst individuals, as discussed in the previous chapter. Identity development, largely thought to grow entirely from adolescence into adulthood, is now understood to start during childhood. Children are aware of their identities through the various systems and messages they receive on a daily basis, consciously and unconsciously. Think about all the messages children hear at school, home, religious communities, via media, through video games, and with peers. The bombardment is astonishing – and children are listening.

Children receive messages all the time about their identities and what outside others perceive and think of those identities. Sometimes this can lead to negative self-image, while other times this can be identity-affirming.

Put yourself in the shoes of a school-based group clinician working on perspective-taking with children ages seven to ten. The group is almost all cisgender boys with one cisgender girl. The girl often wears glittery, sparkly clothes in tones of pink and purple which match her bright personality as do her shoes which are adorned with smiling kittens.

As you practice perspective-taking, you ask the members to physically try on different shoes and guess to whom they might belong. Your shoes are bright pink with smiling kittens on them. You are quick to point out that you think the shoes belong to a girl. The group is equally quick to point out your assumption, reminding you that anybody can wear pink and like kittens, not just girls.

This particular example is used to point out two things:

1 **Identity development has roots in childhood and the seeds which grow in adolescence are planted in the early social messages children receive; and**
2 **It is easy to falsely assume children do not understand their identities so we as clinicians can be careless with our language**.

Child work involves carefully modifying what is effective with adults and tailoring it to children. Children need the same careful articulation of inclusion and openness we provide to adults, but in a developmentally appropriate way. Children are surprisingly perceptive of diversity and difference. They can acutely recognize gendered statements and while they may not understand the broader socialization of gender, similar to other areas of identity they can see experiences relative to gender. Just as adult clinicians move beyond gender-specific statements into the gender continuum, so should child clinicians. As part of our next group activity, we decided to talk about gender using The Genderbread Person, a free online resource talking about the gender continuum (Sam Killermann, www.itspronouncedmetrosexual.com). After prepping caregivers, we talked about sex vs. gender and how each member chooses to express themselves, all within a normalizing framework of exploration. Members used the image as a visual aid to understand themselves and the differences between them. Clinicians can use images such as The Genderbread Person to help children concretize an abstract concept like gender. As with gender described here, **therapists should model openness, inclusion and equity across identities**. We can choose to water the seeds of multiculturalism which grow into awareness and advocacy when we take the cultural opportunities that naturally occur during a group's lifespan (Figure 3.3).

Models of Identity Development

Culturally specific developmental models encompass many areas of identity including racial identity, biracial identity, acculturation, gender, sexual orientation, colonization and morality (D'Andrea, 2014). Overviewing each specific model is beyond the scope of this book. Many models incorporate journeys through awareness, conformity with majority culture and decision-making into advocacy and consideration of one's culture in relation to other cultures. Perhaps the most widely known is Atkinson, Morten, and Sue's (1998) Racial and Cultural Identity Development model, also known as the R/CID model, which is discussed in length

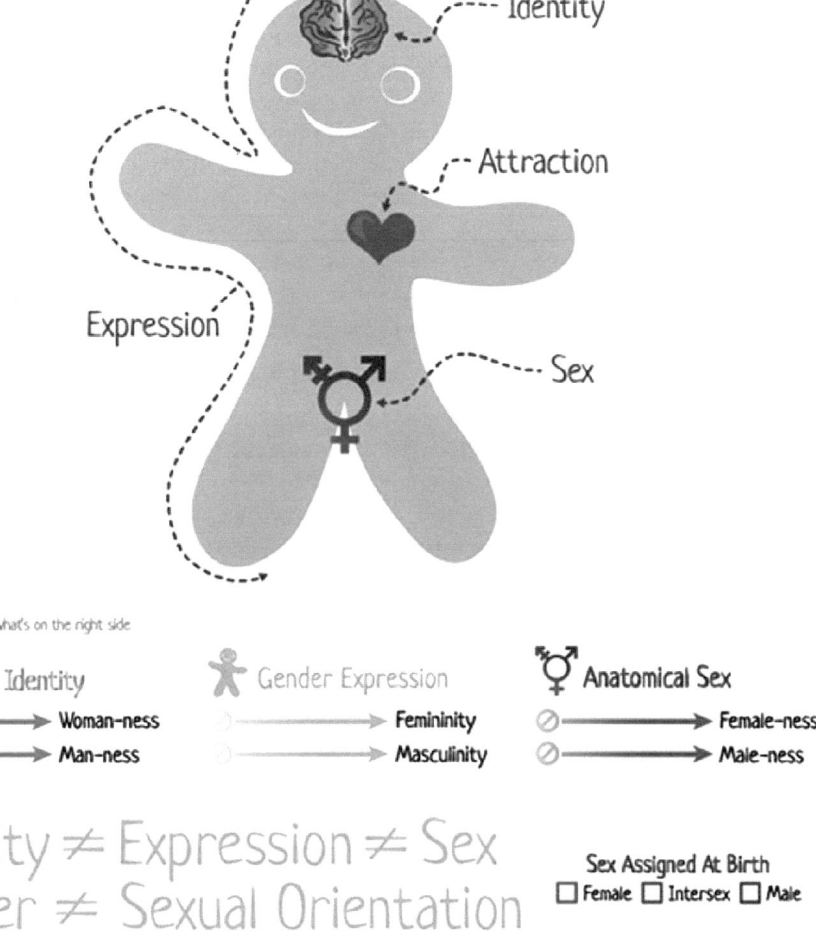

Figure 3.3 The Genderbread Person

in Sue et al.'s (2019) most recent seminal text about multicultural psychological treatment, *Counseling the Culturally Diverse: Theory and Practice*. While it does not fit every client, the R/CID outlines a general framework found in many identity development models:

- Status 1 – **Conformity**: Unequivocal preference for dominant culture over a child's own culture, such as children of color choosing to play with White dolls.
- Status 2 – **Dissonance**: Conflict between a child's preference for their own culture and the dominant culture, potentially seeing positive aspects of their racial identity for the first time, such as dissonance from a Black child seeing stereotypes in Western media.
- Status 3 – **Resistance and Immersion**: Endorsing culture-specific values and rejecting dominant culture entirely, such as a South Korean child only listening to K-pop music and refusing to hear anything else.
- Status 4 – **Introspection**: Development of positive self-identity which may be at odds with the cultural group with more individual consideration of values when making identity decisions, such as a Latinx person having a White friend despite pressure from their cultural group not to.
- Status 5 – **Integrative Awareness**: Commitment to an inner sense of identity and appreciation of their own and other's cultures with a drive to eliminate oppression, such as an ally for LGBTQIA+ attending a Pride march.

While identity development is most pronounced starting in adolescence and into adulthood during one's lifelong, introspective self-journey, children benefit from openly discussing cultural values and norms. **Positive identity shapes resilience** and decreases risky social behavior aimed at inclusion such as gang membership (Ferguson, 2018). **Building resilience is crucial to work with children**. Resilience relates to identity, emotional regulation and social competence. **Group leaders build resilience through positive messages about identity**. Where many children may be shamed for their identities such as a child with ADHD being punished for not sitting still, a trans child chastised for wearing clothing which matches their gender, or a BIPOC child made fun of for the color of their skin, group leaders have a powerful reparative voice through a non-judgmental, encouraging attitude. Affirming statements about a client's identity builds resilience by inspiring ownership and pride over a part of themselves others may actively denigrate. **Simply talking about by identifying and exploring issues of culture, power dynamics, and privilege in child groups sets the stage for positive identity development later in life**.

Mapping development onto culture illuminates many concrete options for talking about culture in child groups. Imagine a tangible game like *identity dominoes* where children sit in a circle and create a physical domino chain of their identities. Using the ADDRESSING model (or another model which encompasses visible and invisible identities), ask children to note their individual identities and choose a domino to represent it. Ask each member about this identity and what it means to them using open-ended questions and statements like "What does it mean to you to be (fill in the blank) or "Tell me what being a kid is like." As you move through each identity, notice and highlight different cultural messages to increase awareness as the domino chain grows longer. Once complete, fill in the gaps of the domino and have each member start the chain reaction from their seat simultaneously. The creation of a chain is an example of both impermanence and connection which illustrates the constantly changing nature of identity. You can even take this a step further in early stages of child groups and ask children to link their dominoes based on their similar identities!

Caregiver-Child Identity Development

Caregivers, parents, extended family, foster parents and broader communities have huge impacts on the cultural identities of children. The environment in which children spend their time is the cultural "air" they breathe. The evidence points in a clear direction for socialization in childhood and how it impacts identity development in adolescence. ***Cultural socialization* refers to cultural messages parents provide and how this is internalized by children, including how they integrate various identities or, for adopted children, understand and integrate messages from their culture of origin** (Lee et al., 2006). Parents adopting children are tasked with identifying and promoting positive identity development through connection with the child's culture of origin.

Racial and ethnic socialization in childhood results in increased self-esteem, academic performance and a more positive Black identity status in adolescence for Black children (Murry et al., 2009). Cultural socialization messages from parents received by Black youth resulted in more positive racial and ethnic identity later in adolescence (Peck et al., 2014). This has implications for culturally homogeneous groups which will be discussed later in the chapter. However, suffice to say that underrepresented populations succeed in environments where the underrepresented identity is seen, valued and promoted, especially with similar peers.

Families, often considered the original group, are also the first point of contact for social and cultural values and communication. In working with Somali, Sierra Leonean, and Nigerian immigrants, Obsiye and Cook (2016) found a heavy family influence on child values including education used for social mobility deeply ingrained in regular social contact. For adoptive Korean-American children, adopting parents were the largest support of ethnic social identity development (Hu et al., 2017). Families are instrumental in how they facilitate identity-related growth.

In short, family values exert a strong influence on childhood beliefs. The more children are allowed to visibly explore their identities and cultures of origin within their childhood environments, the more they are able to develop positive self-identities later in life. Child groups are a unique, powerful way to build such resilience!

Considering all of a client's family, natural environment, socialization history and extended support is a requisite skill for working with children. Children have the difficult job of integrating many different cultural messages. They hear, decipher and slowly mix familial and community values into their budding personalities. They must navigate the complex world of generational identity and, at times, inelegantly combine individual values with dominant culture and family values. **As group leaders, we have the powerful opportunity to promote positive identity development**. The cultural opportunities present in group bring awareness to culture and how it impacts group member's individual experiences and the group as a whole. Affirmations of group differences promote a sense of pride for various identities and sets the stage for advocacy later in life.

Creating Brave Spaces

If affirmations create pride and slowly build resilience, the opposite is true for intentional and unintentional shaming experiences between group members. Like any group, child groups represent a social microcosm where they bring in their own biases which show up in member-to-member interactions. When a group member is allowed to emotionally harm another group member, even unintentionally, the group as a whole will likely struggle to engage due to lack of safety. Cohesive groups make room for process interactions between members which build relationships and are naturally healing. Group members can then internalize the safety found inside the group. **Internalized safety leads to the establishment of a *brave space*, or an emotional space within the group to process difficult topics including personal struggles, social justice issues and diversity within the group and larger**

societal contexts (Ali, 2017; Arao & Clemens, 2013). This idea relates to the intrapsychic safety individual members feel on when vulnerability and self-expression are valued and cultivated within a group. When in a brave space, members are more willing to actively discuss social justice issues and identity development.

The idea of a brave space originated with college students but is directly applicable to child groups. Theoretically, the concept makes logical sense with current research regarding how **safety in groups relates to the group's overall cultural openness** (Kivlighan et al., 2020). Children bring into group their family cultural experiences which to them are normal experiences and which they inherently believe are universal to others. The relativistic nature of normalcy means children are often confused by differing personal and family practices explored in the richness of group process. **By compassionately exploring the inherent differences between members using group process rather than simply moving through content, child groups create brave spaces**.

Imagine the following dyadic interaction between two group members while they are working on treasure maps (a goal-setting activity):

RAFIQ (nine-year-old, second-generation, cisgender, Iranian-American male): "I like your treasure map, Kelly. I'm hungry. What are you eating tonight? Mother is making adas polo and my belly is hungry NOW! Do you like adas polo?"

KELLY (11-year-old, fourth-generation, cisgender, Irish-American female): "I don't know, probably like chicken nuggets I guess. We like always eat chicken nuggets after group. It's our Wednesday thing. What did you say you were gonna eat? 'Das' what?!"

RAFIQ: "Chicken nuggets? You eat them every week? I am going to eat A-D-A-S, P-O-L-O. Adas polo. It's my favorite."

KELLY (looking confused): "What IS A-D-S, P-L-O-O?"

RAFIQ: "It's like beans and rice and stuff. Mother makes the BEST adas polo."

KELLY: "Is there any chicken in it?"

RAFIQ: "BLECH (makes retching noise)! My family does NOT eat chicken."

KELLY (looking surprised with wide eyes): "NO CHICKEN?! Then how do you eat chicken nuggets? What about hamburgers?"

RAFIQ: "DOUBLE BLECH. I don't eat chicken nuggets. Or hamburgers. Hamburgers are animals! We don't eat animals. Father says we must respect life all the time, even when we eat."

KELLY: (looking aghast) "NO CHICKEN NUGGETS?! I think I would DIE. Your family is weird."

RAFIQ (cheeks flushed, starting to get angry): "My family isn't weird, YOU'RE WEIRD! Just SHUT UP!" (Rafiq looks embarrassed and puts down his crayon)

This is a cultural opportunity for this specific dyad. As a therapist, how would you respond in a way which exemplifies openness? Kelly and Rafiq experience different food-related norms in their households relative to family identities and values.

An affirming response would include some of the following features:

- Providing conflict resolution to help Kelly and Rafiq calmly exchange perspectives and listen to each other before they escalate;
- Processing Rafiq's feelings, especially about Kelly's microaggression;
- Processing Kelly's feelings, especially about the end of the interaction;
- Encouraging openness from both members;
- Exploring reasons for Kelly and Rafiq's diets with a curious and humble attitude;
- Normalizing individual differences;

- Problem-solving language to use in future interactions about differences; and
- Modeling acceptance of each other without judgment.

Taking this cultural opportunity allows Kelly and Rafiq to deepen their individual relationship while exemplifying a typical child interaction. The reality is, in any group, interactions such as this one happen all the time. Part of group leadership with children is making sure these moments do not pass without attention. Skipping Rafiq's hurt feelings from Kelly's microaggression would send messages to Rafiq that the group is unsafe for him, that he cannot talk about his family or their choices, and that group leaders will not protect him from emotional injury. The same is true in responding to Kelly. Group leaders can help Kelly understand the hurtful nature of her words and how she can learn about others by expressing curiosity without judgment. Teaching and responding to Kelly in this way also reinforces the idea that the group as a whole can make mistakes and talk about difficult subjects without shaming. Groupwork with children is built upon many of these exchanges, positive and negative. By resolving conflict and encouraging discussion of cultural differences, children feel a sense of safety to explore themselves and more fully experience the healing power of group therapy.

Group Composition: Homogeneous vs. Heterogeneous Groups and Cultural Adaptations for Specific Groups

Group composition is a highly subjective task for group therapists. There is no right or wrong way to achieve this, other than that group clinicians must be intentional with the group they would like to create. At times, homogenous groups are an important avenue for connection and specific therapeutic work, such as a group for children on the autism spectrum. The homogenous group has the opportunity to richly and deeply explore a certain identity. Conversely, a mixed-gender, -grade and -diagnostic group can provide a learning environment which may imitate the diversity in their natural environments. The heterogeneous group has the opportunity to learn about diversity between members and skills which can be used outside of group. Both have important roles based on the setting where they occur. **When planning groups, intentionality is key**.

Group composition will be discussed in greater depth in Chapters 6 and 7. However, one area for discussion here is the idea of constructing culture-specific and culturally adapted groups. In the psychological literature, assessments and therapy are predominantly normed through the dominant culture and then subsequently applied to various sub- and non-dominant cultures.

Honoring Children, Mending the Circle (HC-MC) (Bigfoot & Schmidt, 2006) is an example of a Trauma-Focused Cognitive-Behavioral Therapy (TF-CBT) approach culturally modified specifically for indigenous cultures in North America including American Indians and Alaskan Natives. HC-MC takes several cultural beliefs from North American indigenous cultures such as interconnection, the spirituality of all things and the dynamism of existence and overlays them on TF-CBT to modify interventions in a way which honors culture (Bigfoot & Schmidt, 2010). Instead of a trauma narrative with just the clinician and clients, the group as a whole might decide with their families the medium in which to express the narrative including a written story, dance or journey stick. Programs such as HC-MC are an exemplary way to create culturally focused homogenous groups. There are many different ways to center a group around a specific identity.

In creating homogeneous spaces surrounding an identity, positive identity development is paramount. Positive identity development is easily reinforced in such homogeneous groups which increases therapeutic outcomes, seen in Steen's work with African American elementary school children (2009) or Malott and Paone's book titled *Group Activities for Latino/a Youth: Strengthening Identities and Resilience Through Counseling* (2016). Homogenous groups surrounding a particular identity are typically led by a leader who shares that identity which also fosters positive development through modeling. Creating culture-specific homogenous groups or using cultural adaptations are excellent ways to make accessible, relevant group therapy for children. In locations with a high cultural affiliation or population, such groups can be incredibly powerful. Whether homogeneous or heterogeneous groups, it is the clinician's job to take a cultural humility standpoint in order to learn about populations with which they are unfamiliar and integrate those pieces into child groups, even if for just one group member.

Many of the culturally adapted and culturally focused groups have several things in common:

1   The *blending of cultural practices and beliefs with an established theoretical framework* helps create best practices for specific populations and scenarios.
2   An emphasis on *positive identity development* related to a specific identity.
3   *Modification of interventions* directly related to the cultural practices of a specific group.

Steen and Bauman (2009) discuss through their video series the power of leading multicultural groups with diverse members. **No matter what the age, it is developmentally appropriate to talk about identity** in ways which also honors the cognitive and social development of those within the group. Most clinicians run groups with diverse clients and many distinct identities. Heterogeneous groups provide a social microcosm for child clients which can introduce them to cross-cultural socialization. Heterogeneous groups allow for the unique experience of talking about different cultures and identities that children bring. While homogenous groups bring strength through connection over a particular culture, heterogeneous groups bring strength through individuality and uniqueness amongst members which can be shared for the enrichment of group processes. Both provide distinct avenues of effective treatment by overlapping culture on group structure. In the group development phase, consider whether a homogeneous or heterogeneous group would be most effective for the group you are creating!

Discussion Questions

1   What are some of the major ADDRESSING populations in your area?
2   How might you alter your own practice, learn more about a specific culture or partner with an agency helping an underserved population to create a group specifically for a non-dominant population in your area?
3   How might cultural adaptations to group therapy impact the perception of mental health within those populations?

Handling Microaggressions in Groups with Children

Microaggressions **are a common-place, brief, often-subtle form of stereotyping and discrimination which have harmful impact on the target person or group of persons** (Sue et al., 2007). Originally formulated by Pierce (1974) relative to Black Americans, microaggressions were later expanded upon by Rowe (1974) to include all marginalized groups. Atkinson, Morten, and Sue's (1998) further break down microaggressions into three different types:

- ***Microassaults*** are direct, overt insults purposefully chosen to convey harm and discrimination towards a particular identity. **Children learn from their environments, and this includes discriminatory behavior**. Children may direct racial slurs at other group members with intent to cause harm after hearing the term in their natural environment.

- ***Microinsults*** are unintentional comments which are insensitive to a layer of someone's identity. For example, one child in a group might ask an Asian-American group member for help on their math homework which conveys the stereotype that all Asian people excel at math. A cisgender boy in group may not want to talk about feelings because "only girls do that," showing a socially constructed, gendered approach to roles and related behaviors which is demeaning towards girls and women.

- ***Microinvalidations*** are comments or actions which invalidate the experiences of a target person or group. A group member with cerebral palsy may be talking about how bad they feel on a certain day including how difficult it is to get out of bed. Another group member may invalidate that experience by making a comment such as "What's so hard about getting out of bed?" In the example earlier in the chapter about Ramadan, a Christian group member could make statements which invalidate the Muslim group member's lack of positive religious experiences in their school. Statements such as "we always celebrate Christmas at my school" or "maybe you should do a different holiday so the school will celebrate with you" can be motivated by kindness or connection but be experienced as insulting. **Microinvalidations are particularly common with children given their egocentric worldview**. Perspective-taking activities build empathy for different identities and their experiences.

Handling microaggressions in groups is a core example of process work. Microaggressions are often unintentional. Processing the impact of the individual statement on the target group member allows for awareness of the microaggression itself and creates a sense of safety to discuss issues of identity. Processing with child groups may be playful or serious based on the content.

During process work with children, technical aids are helpful. The remote control used in Chapter 2 on developmental psychology for child groups is an excellent example, as it can be used to "fast-forward," "pause," "rewind," or "play" a group interaction. For example, it could "pause" the group in the middle of an activity to encourage all members to freeze in place. Then, the member targeted by the microaggression could be allowed to "play" by talking about their feelings in reaction to the microaggression while the rest of the group listens. The group leader can "rewind" the microaggressing member to work with the group to find an earlier statement in the group which matches intent and impact. This brings in the member who was targeted to allow a repairing interaction to occur. It also allows the group leader(s) to provide scaffolding or psychoeducation about why such statements are harmful. Once a solution is identified, the group leader can press "play" on the remote control to rehearse the new statement and see its impact.

Dyadic work between child members facilitates a reparative effect which also signals to the group that it is safe to talk about issues of diversity. Once clarified, the dyad can decide to press "play" on the rest of the group to continue the activity. Process moments increase group sensitivity to diversity and also model how to handle microaggressions in their daily lives.

Successfully handling microaggressions may not be as important as the overall comfort of a group's ability to talk openly about culture (Hook et al., 2016; Kivlighan et al., 2020). **A group's overall comfort is closely tied to the leader's acceptance and comfort**

of minority group members (Meeussen et al., 2014). Child group leaders can greatly impact identity development by creating safe, brave group cultures which allow members to talk about all areas of their individual experiences.

Microaffirmations

Mary Rowe coined the terms microaffirmations and microinequities starting in the 1970s. During that era, the discussion about microinequities helped develop the more modern concept of microaggressions by talking about how individuals can unconsciously or unintentionally harm somebody they perceive to be different. On the other hand, microaffirmations are a way to actively encourage positive cultural development. ***Microaffirmations*** (Rowe, 2008) **are small, subtle acts which happen publicly and privately and occur when people help others succeed**. Researchers are just beginning to identify types of microaffirmations and how or why they are critical in developing positive identity and racial climates (Pérez Huber et al., 2021; Rolón-Dow, 2019; Rolón-Dow & Davison, 2020). Microaffirmations intentionally disrupt marginalization by directly challenging stereotypes and negative cultural messages perceived from the majority culture. They have the potential to promote increased health and academic outcomes for underrepresented populations, but research on this is currently limited. Applying this concept to children provides a clear direction for promoting cultural self-efficacy. Simply talking about and encouraging children's various identities can provide an affirming atmosphere. Therapy, and group therapy in particular, provides a unique avenue through which clinicians can greatly impact child cultural development. Examples of microaffirmations include:

- Affirming, diverse media and books in the office waiting room;
- Intentionally reminding clients of strengths which defy stereotypes;
- Recognizing and discussing the positive impacts of one's identity;
- Celebrating holidays relevant to different cultures during group;
- Validating the experiences of group members, including microaggressions inside and outside of group.

Exercise

Imagine the following scenario between two group members and a leader. Put yourself in the shoes of the group leader. First, identify some of the microaggressions and evaluate the efficacy of the leader's responses.

GROUP LEADER: "Alright, we have a new person joining group today. Emerson, can you tell us a little bit about yourself? We have some questions written on the board: Name, Age, Pronouns, Why You're in Group, Favorite Food, and Favorite Place."

EMERSON: "My name is Emerson, I am 12 years old, my pronouns are they/them…"

KAELIN (cisgender male, 11 years old): "What do you mean they and them? You look like a girl to me."

EMERSON (looking embarrassed): "I don't always feel like a girl, and gender is just a label. People get to choose their gender. I choose they/them."

KAELIN: "That doesn't make sense. You look like a girl. You ARE a girl. My dad says if you look and dress like a girl or a guy, then you're a girl or a guy. Period. Maybe you should be a girl. You won't make friends if you don't. Not with me."

EMERSON (looking uncomfortable): "…"

GROUP LEADER: "Kaelin, please stop interrupting Emerson. Emerson, please continue."

EMERSON: "My favorite food is saag paneer. My favorite place is the forest by my house. I climb trees there a lot."

KAELIN: "Girls can't climb trees good. Did somebody teach you to climb them?"

GROUP LEADER: "Kaelin, please do not interrupt Emerson again. Emerson, I want you to know that girls are great at climbing trees, just like boys."

KAELIN: "But…"

GROUP LEADER: "Kaelin, it is not your turn right now. Please listen. Now, who wants to go next with their introductions?"

Mistakes are helpful ways to learn, and therapy is no exception. Given the complexity and speed of interactions, group clinicians often miss the opportunity to address microaggressions. In the above vignette, the group leader did little to curb the microaggressions in the interaction. Kaelin stated a microinvalidation, microassault and microinsult directed towards Emerson. Kaelin's statement about Emerson not making friends could be considered a microassault as he is communicating he will not be friends with Emerson because of this identity. Kaelin saying girls cannot climb trees is a microinsult. Lastly, Kaelin viewing Emerson as a girl despite her identification of they/them pronouns is a microinvalidation.

If you were the leader, how could you respond to Emerson and Kaelin's interaction to make Emerson feel welcome and establish the importance of respect within this group? How do you feel Emerson is likely to feel during this interaction? When microaggressions go unchecked during sessions, groups feel unsafe. Members who are targets of microaggressions can internalize messages, leading to negative perceptions of themselves. If you were the group leader, how would you manage this conflict? Additionally, how could you use microaffirmations to help Emerson feel secure within this group?

Staying Up-To-Date with Language

Language matters. Language facilitates our understanding of the world. With increasing research relative to identity and the dynamics of power and privilege, part of the call to action for therapists is to learn and maintain flexibility with trends in language. Language changes over time, evident in even dictionaries changing and eliminating words (take a look at when "selfie" formally entered the dictionary). Over time, targeted populations often "take back" slurs and turn them into words of power to disarm their insulting nature. For example, the word "queer" was once used as a homophobic slur and is now commonly seen as a term for somebody questioning their sexuality. The term "fat" is often used as a slur against people with larger bodies. However, just like the word "queer," "fat" is being reclaimed to reduce anti-fat bias and shaming.

Children and adolescents are particularly sensitive to clinician language which denotes the clinician's understanding of diversity issues and concurrently, how safe it is to talk about identity. Subtle language cues and tests provide feedback to clients about the safety within group spaces. **Listen to your clients and how they identify themselves**. We all want to be seen and validated for our identities. They shape, form and challenge us over time in relation to ourselves, our history and other people and cultures. Using our client's language not only shows we are listening; it shows that we see our clients for who they are.

The language surrounding particular identities shifts over time and our job as clinicians is to flexibly shift with them to best serve our clients. Nothing else validates clients like reflecting their experiences and identities. This by proxy is paramount to the therapeutic alliance, creation of safety and group cohesion.

Language shapes how we perceive and understand the world around us. Websites such as racialequitytools.org/glossary, hrc.org/resources/glossary-of-terms, LGBTQhealth.ca and dictionary.apa.org offer up-to-date resources about identity and multiculturalism. They are tools clinicians can use to stay current, inclusive and equitable in language and practice. Appendix A includes a current list of terms (as of this publication date) which may be helpful. Chances are good that within a few years or even months, some of these terms will be outdated. Please use it as a starting point with the caveat that language and how we use it is constantly shifting!

Summary

The growing body of research on the diversity of human experiences is a call to action for clinicians. Child group clinicians are uniquely positioned to empathically encourage identity development through cultural humility and a multicultural orientation. Children's understanding of abstract traditions and self-identity are rooted in early-life experiences which are explored and integrated during adolescence and beyond. If left unexplored, children are most likely to interpret the cultural messages of the dominant group which, especially for those in underrepresented populations, can be discouraging, shameful and outright harming. Attention to diversity, marginalization and privilege plants the seeds, tills the soil and waters the earth in service of positive self-identities. Children, some of the most vulnerable among us, are owed that justice and respect.

We must intentionally honor and work with our child client's cultures and include them to enrich our group spaces. Children, just like the clinicians leading their groups, can learn vastly differing perspectives which enrich their perspectives, lives and worldviews. **As clinicians with children, we must doubly encourage openness, curiosity, flexibility, compassion and courage while discussing the many complexities of power and privilege**. Open ears and an open heart provide ample opportunity for healing and growth.

References

Ali, D. (2017). NASPA Policy and Practice Series: Safe Spaces and Brave Spaces, Historical Contexts and Recommendations for Student Affairs Professionals. Retrieved February 26, 2021, from https://www.naspa.org/images/uploads/main/Policy_and_Practice_No_2_Safe_Brave_Spaces.pdf

American Psychological Association. (2003). Guidelines on multicultural education, training, research, practice, and organizational change for psychologists. *American Psychologist, 58,* 377–402.

American Psychological Association. (2017). Multicultural Guidelines: An Ecological Approach to Context, Identity, and Intersectionality. Retrieved from: https://www.apa.org/about/policy/multicultural-guidelines.pdf

Arao, B., & Clemens, K. (2013). From safe spaces to brave spaces: a new way to frame dialogue around diversity and social justice. In L. Landreman (Ed.), *The art of effective facilitation: Reflections from social justice educators* (pp. 135–150). Sterling, VA: Stylus Publishing.

Atkinson, D. R., Morten, G., & Sue, D. W. (1998). *Counseling American minorities: A cross-cultural perspective* (5th ed.). Boston, MA: McGraw-Hill.

BigFoot, D. S., & Schmidt, S. R. (2006). *Honoring children, mending the circle (trauma-focused cognitive-behavior therapy)*. Oklahoma City: Indian Country Child Trauma Center, University of Oklahoma Health Sciences Center.

BigFoot, D. S., & Schmidt, S. R. (2010). Honoring children, mending the circle: cultural adaptation of trauma-focused cognitive-behavioral therapy for American Indian and Alaska native children. *Journal of clinical psychology, 66*(8), 847–856. https://doi.org/10.1002/jclp.20707

Bronfenbrenner, U. (1979). *The ecology of human development.* Cambridge, MA: Harvard University Press.

Carter, S. E., Ong, M. L., Simons, R. L., Gibbons, F. X., Lei, M. K., & Beach, S. R. H. (2019). The effect of early discrimination on accelerated aging among African Americans. *Health Psychology, 38*(11), 1010–1013. https://doi.org/10.1037/hea0000788

Chung, R. C.-Y., Bemak, F., Talleyrand, R. M., & Williams, J. M. (2018). Challenges in promoting race dialogues in psychology training: Race and gender perspectives. *The Counseling Psychologist, 46*(2), 213–240. https://doi.org/10.1177/0011000018758262

Clauss-Ehlers, C., Chiriboga, D., Hunter, S., Roysircar, G., & Tummala-Narra, P. (2019). APA multicultural guidelines executive summary: Ecological Approach to context, identity, and intersectionality. *American Psychologist, 74*, 232–244.

Crenshaw, K., & Bonis, O. (2005). Mapping the margins: Intersectionality, identity politics, and violence against women of color. *Cahiers du Genre, 2*(2), 51–82. https://doi.org/10.3917/cdge.039.0051

Davis, D. E., DeBlaere, C., Brubaker, K., Owen, J., Jordan, T. A. II, Hook, J. N., & Van Tongeren, D. R. (2016). Microaggressions and perceptions of cultural humility in counseling. *Journal of Counseling & Development, 94*(4), 483–493. https://doi.org/10.1002/jcad.12107

D'Andrea, M. (2014). Understanding racial/cultural identity development theories to promote effective multicultural group counseling. In J. L. DeLucia-Waack, C. R. Kalodner, & M. T. Riva (Eds.), *Handbook of group counseling and psychotherapy* (pp. 196–208). Thousand Oaks, CA: Sage Publications, Inc. https://doi.org/10.4135/9781544308555.n15

DiAngelo, R. (2011). White fragility. *International Journal of Critical Pedagogy, 3*(3), 54–70.

Ferguson, L. (2018). 'Could an increased focus on identity development in the provision of children's services help shape positive outcomes for care leavers?' A literature review. *Child Care in Practice, 24*(1), 76–91. https://doi.org/10.1080/13575279.2016.1199536

Fivush, R., & Wang, Q. (2005) Emotion talk in mother-child conversations of the shared past: the effects of culture, gender, and event valence. *Journal of Cognition and Development, 6*(4), 489–506, https://doi.org/10.1207/s15327647jcd0604_3

Hays, P. A. (2001). *Addressing cultural complexities in practice: A framework for clinicians and counselors.* Washington, DC: American Psychological Association.

Hays, P. A. (2016). *Addressing cultural complexities in practice: Assessment, diagnosis, and therapy* (3rd ed.). Washington, DC: American Psychological Association. https://doi.org/10.1037/14801-000

Henrich, J., Heine, S. J., & Norenzayan, A. (2010). The weirdest people in the world? *Behavioral and Brain Sciences, 33*(2–3), 61–83. https://doi.org/10.1017/S0140525X0999152X

Hook, J. N., Farrell, J. E., Davis, D. E., DeBlaere, C., Van Tongeren, D. R., & Utsey, S. O. (2016). Cultural humility and racial microaggressions in counseling. *Journal of Counseling Psychology, 63*(3), 269–277. https://doi.org/10.1037/cou0000114

Hook, J., Davis, D., Owen, J., & DeBlaere, C. (2017). *Cultural humility: Engaging diverse identities in therapy.* Washington, DC: American Psychological Association.

Hu, A. W., Zhou, X., & Lee, R. M. (2017). Ethnic socialization and ethnic identity development among internationally adopted Korean American adolescents: A seven-year follow-up. *Developmental Psychology, 53*(11), 2066–2077. https://doi.org/10.1037/dev0000421

Kaklauskas, F. J., & Greene, L. R. (Eds.). (2019). *Core principles of group psychotherapy: An integrated theory, research, and practice training manual* (1st ed.). New York: Routledge. https://doi.org/10.4324/9780429260803

Kendi, D. I. X. (2016). *Stamped from the beginning.* New York: Avalon Publishing Group.

Kernahan, C., & Davis, T. (2010). What are the long-term effects of learning about racism? *Teaching of Psychology, 37*(1), 41–45. https://doi.org/10.1080/00986280903425748

Killermann, S. (n.d.). Breaking through the binary: Gender explained using continuums. https://www.itspronouncedmetrosexual.com/2011/11/breaking-through-the-binary-gender-explained-using-continuums/

Kivlighan, D. M. III, Swancy, A. G., Smith, E., & Brennaman, C. (2020). Examining racial microaggressions in group therapy and the buffering role of members' perceptions of their group's multicultural orientation. *Journal of Counseling Psychology.* Advance online publication. https://doi.org/10.1037/cou0000531

Lee, R. M., Grotevant, H. D., Hellerstedt, W. L., Gunnar, M. R., & Minnesota International Adaption Project Team. (2006). Cultural socialization in families with internationally adopted children. *Journal* of family psychology: *Journal of the Division of Family Psychology of the American Psychological Association (Division 43)*, *20*(4), 571–580. https://doi.org/10.1037/0893-3200.20.4.571

Malott, K. M., & Paone, T. R. (Eds.). (2016). *Group Activities for Latino/a Youth: Strengthening Identities and Resiliencies through Counseling* (1st ed.). New York: Routledge. https://doi.org/10.4324/9781315751481

Meeussen, L., Otten, S., & Phalet, K. (2014). Managing diversity: How leaders' multiculturalism and colorblindness affect work group functioning. *Group Processes & Intergroup Relations*, *17*(5), 629–644. https://doi.org/10.1177/1368430214525809

Murry, V. M., Berkel, C., Brody, G. H., Miller, S. J., & Chen, Y. -f. (2009). Linking parental socialization to interpersonal protective processes, academic self-presentation, and expectations among rural African American youth. *Cultural Diversity and Ethnic Minority Psychology*, *15*(1), 1–10. https://doi.org/10.1037/a0013180

National Association of Social Workers. (2015). *Standards and indicators for cultural competence in social work practice*. Washington, DC: NASW.

National Child Welfare Workforce Institute. (n.d.). Cultural Humility Practice Principles. Retrieved April 17, 2021, from https://ncwwi.org/index.php/resourcemenu/resource-library/inclusivity-racial-equity/cultural-responsiveness/1415-cultural-humility-practice-principles/file

Obsiye, M., & Cook, R. (2016). Forum: Cultural identity and (dis)continuities of children of immigrant communities. *Cultural Studies of Science Education*, *11*(4), 1061–1070.

Peck, S. C., Brodish, A. B., Malanchuk, O., Banerjee, M., & Eccles, J. S. (2014). Racial/ethnic socialization and identity development in black families: The role of parent and youth reports. *Developmental Psychology*, *50*(7), 1897–1909. https://doi.org/10.1037/a0036800

Pérez Huber, L, Gonzalez, T., Robles, G., & Solórzano D.G. (2021). Racial microaffirmations as a response to racial microaggressions: Exploring risk and protective factors. *New Ideas in Psychology (63)*, Article 100880. https://doi.org/10.1016/j.newideapsych.2021.100880

Pierce, C. M. (1974). Psychiatric problems of the black minority. In S. Arieti (Ed.), *American Handbook of Psychiatry* (pp. 512–523). New York: Basic Books.

Ratts, M. J., Singh, A. A., Nassar-McMillan, S., Butler, S. K., & McCullough, J. R. (2016). Multicultural and social justice counseling competencies: Guidelines for the counseling profession. *Journal of Multicultural Counseling and Development*, *44*(1), 28–48.

Rolón-Dow, R. (2019). Stories of microaggressions and microaffirmations: A framework for listening to campus racial climate. *Currents*, *1*(1), 64–78. http://dx.doi.org/10.3998/currents.17387731.0001.106

Rolón-Dow, R., & Davison, A. (2020). Theorizing racial microaffirmations: A Critical Race/LatCrit approach. *Ethnicity and Education*, *24*(2), 245–261. https://doi.org/10.1080/13613324.2020.1798381

Rowe. M. (1974). Saturn's Rings: A study of the minutiae of sexism which maintain discrimination and inhibit affirmative action results in corporations and non-profit institutions. In *Graduate and Professional Education of Women* (pp. 1–9). Washington, DC: American Association of University Women.

Rowe, M. (2008). Micro-affirmation and Micro-inequalities. *Journal of the International Ombudsman Association*, *1*(1), 45–48.

Sommarö, S., Andersson, A., & Skagerström, J. (2020). A deviation too many? Healthcare professionals' knowledge and attitudes concerning patients with intellectual disability disrupting norms regarding sexual orientation and/or gender identity. *Journal of Applied Research in Intellectual Disabilities*, *33*(6), 1199–1209. https://doi.org/10.1111/jar.12739

Steen, S. (2009). Group counseling for African American elementary students: An exploratory study. *The Journal for Specialists in Group Work*, *34*, 101–117.

Steen, S., & Bauman, S. (2009). Celebrating Diversity: Leading Multicultural Groups. Psychotherapy. net Productions. Available at: https://www.psychotherapy.net/video/diversity-group-children

Sue, D. W., Bucceri, J., Lin, A. I., Nadal, K. L., & Torino, G. C. (2007). Racial microaggressions and the Asian American experience. *Cultural Diversity and Ethnic Minority Psychology*, *13*(1), 72–81. https://doi.org/10.1037/1099-9809.13.1.72

Sue, D. W., Sue, D., Neville, H. A., & Smith, L. (2019). *Counseling the culturally diverse: Theory and practice* (8th ed.). Hoboken, NJ: Wiley.

Swanson, D. P., Spencer, M. B., Harpalani, V., Dupree, D., Noll, E., Ginzburg, S., & Seaton, G. (2003). Psychosocial Development in Racially and Ethnically Diverse Youth: Conceptual and Methodological Challenges in the 21st Century. Retrieved from http://repository.upenn.edu/gse_pubs/2

Tervalon, M., & Murray-García, J. (1998). Cultural humility versus cultural competence: A critical distinction in defining physician training outcomes in multicultural education. *Journal of Health Care for the Poor and Underserved, 9*(2), 117–125. https://doi.org/10.1353/hpu.2010.0233

Torres, H. J. (2016). On the margins: The depiction of Muslims in young children's Picturebooks. *Children's Literature in Education, 47*(3), 191–208.

Turban, J. L., & Ehrensaft, D. (2018). Research review: Gender identity in youth: treatment paradigms and controversies. *Journal of Child Psychology & Psychiatry, 59*(12), 1228–1243. https://doi.org/10.1111/jcpp.12833

Waters, A., & Asbill, L. (2013). Reflections on cultural humility. CYF News. http://www.apa.org/pi/families/resources/newsletter/2013/08/cultural-humility

4 Interpersonal Theoretical Foundations

Tony L. Sheppard

Introduction

Advances in neuroscience offer support for the long-held belief that development in the areas of cognition, emotional functioning, identity formation and other key areas of self-identification and self-regulation occur in the context of significant relationships. Siegel (2020) asserts that some aspects of our development are "experience-dependent." He promotes **the foundational idea that our interpersonal experiences shape who we become with regard to our abilities to connect, remain in relationship and to self-regulate**. Understanding such processes allows us to more fully identify and utilize the interactional aspects of group therapy.

The foundation of any therapeutic work with children is the growth of developmentally appropriate self-management abilities. Children come to therapy with a need to improve their ability to utilize available environmental and internal resources to better manage the situations in their lives. Whether this focuses on management of emotion, behavior or the world of peers, the purpose of most group psychotherapy with children is to support them in developing effective self-regulation capabilities. **Neurobiology increasingly points in the direction of interpersonal processes as the key to developing self-regulation**. Regulation of cognition and emotion is central to a child's ability to connect with others and thereby begin to define themselves. When children fail to acquire the ability to form relationships with others, most developmental models predict poor outcomes in many realms. Group therapy with children must seek to assist them in developing the ability to initiate and maintain healthy relationships.

As a starting point for considering adaptive interpersonal abilities, a metaphor that captures the ideal is found in the work of Gershen Kaufman (1992). Kaufman describes the *interpersonal bridge* as "the bond which ties two individuals together…becomes a vehicle to facilitate mutual understanding, growth, and change" (p. 12). When the interpersonal nature of learning and development is considered, the importance of interpersonal connection becomes evident. In other words, human beings need connections with other human beings in order to learn and develop most effectively. This metaphor of a bridge that connects people offers the group therapist a sense of the goal in creating an environment where learning and development can occur. A necessary component of group work with children, then, is assisting them in connecting with adults and with each other. Often, this flows from the aforementioned work on self-regulation. In fact, **there is a recursive and reciprocal relationship between self-regulation and healthy relationships**. The formation of the interpersonal bridge is both a product of and a necessary ingredient for good self-regulatory abilities in children (Siegel, 2020).

DOI: 10.4324/9781003189701-4

The field of interpersonal neurobiology offers insights into how we connect with others. This has implications for group therapy with children. Building upon self-regulatory capacity, an equally important goal in children's groups is to develop social/emotional expression abilities and to help children form meaningful connections with each other. This, then, serves as a template for the establishment of other relationships in their lives. The combination of self-regulatory capacity and the ability to appropriately and accurately express oneself emotionally serve as the building blocks for healthy relationships.

Whether the focus of a group is depression, disruptive behavior, low self-esteem, anxiety, trauma or other presenting problems, the learning of self-regulatory skills in an interpersonal context is foundational. The ultimate goal of any therapy group is to facilitate members' ability to form meaningful relationships with others and a prerequisite for this is an ability to regulate the self. This chapter features a clinical vignette, the purpose of which is to demonstrate key components. The use of an interpersonal process foundation best facilitates the acquisition of self-regulatory capacities in the service of forming meaningful relationships. It is important to note that these process elements of a group are operating whether or not they become an overt focus of the group. The child group therapist is cautioned that they ignore these interpersonal process elements to the detriment of their groups. As Yalom and Leszcz (2020) state so aptly, "The process focus is the power cell of the group" (p. 194).

Since the quality of relationships in the group setting is of great importance, this chapter deals with qualities of the therapist and their involvement in the group that are conducive to this work. **In an interpersonal context, the group psychotherapist utilizes their own involvement, interaction and presence in the sessions to bring about change**. Therefore, a discussion of therapist qualities and the issue of countertransference is essential. Haen (writing in Haen & Aronson, 2017) notes that integrative approaches are critical to working with youth. He suggests that the child and adolescent group therapist might employ a vast array of interventions such as cognitive behavioral therapy, expressive art approaches, play-based approaches and many others. It should be noted that maintaining an interpersonal process focus does not preclude the use of these interventions.

Therapeutic Factors

It is critical that the child group therapist consider what makes groups effective. While focused on group work with adults, Yalom and Leszcz's 11 curative factors of group have formed the foundation of what we know about therapeutic factors in groups (Yalom & Leszcz, 2020). The following table lists the 11 therapeutic factors with a brief description of each.

A number of authors have noted the paucity of research into mechanisms of therapeutic action in children's groups (Haen, in Haen & Aronson, 2017; Shechtman, 2007, in Haen & Aronson, 2017). Despite this, there is some research and a great deal of clinical wisdom that sheds light on these change agents in working with children in groups (Schectman, 2007). In fact, much of the existing research in this area has been done with adolescents, so the child group therapist is left to assume that similar processes are at work in child groups. Shechtman et al. (2007) found the three most-relevant therapeutic factors in adolescent groups to be Group Cohesiveness, Catharsis and Development of socializing techniques. Shechtman (2007) cites Corder, Whiteside and Haizlip (1981) who found the following factors to be most effective in groups with adolescents: Self-disclosure/catharsis, interpersonal learning, group cohesiveness and support, hope and helping others. Finally, Aronson (writing in Haen & Aronson, 2017) notes the importance of a number of therapeutic factors in work with youth including: Universality, imparting information, recapitulation of the family experience, altruism, socializing

Table 4.1 Yalom's 11 Therapeutic Factors

Therapeutic Factor	Brief Description
Instillation of Hope	Creation of positive expectation for change
Universality	Understanding that many problems are shared by others/"We're all in the same boat"
Imparting Information	Sharing didactic instruction about mental health, the group or giving advice, suggestions or direct guidance
Altruism	Creating a sense that one is helpful to others
The Corrective Recapitulation of the Primary Family Group	Interacting in ways that resemble the client's primary family experience in a manner that is corrective
Development of Socializing Techniques	Helping members to acquire new interpersonal skills and strategies
Imitative Behavior	Observational learning that occurs as others struggle, grow, and change in the group
Interpersonal Learning	Group therapy analog of insight, working through transference and the corrective emotional experience in individual therapy (Yalom & Leszcz, 2020, p. 33)
Group Cohesiveness	Group therapy analog to the relationship in individual therapy (Yalom & Leszcz, p. 73)
Catharsis	Expression of emotion/Getting things off one's chest
Existential Factors	Confronting things that have to do with the "Human Condition"

techniques, instilling a sense of hope and learning the importance of interpersonal relationships (p. 3). Frequently, these insights are based upon asking participants in the groups what they found helpful. Unfortunately, the research that assesses what group members rate as therapeutic is quite variable across groups, depending on type of group, client characteristics, therapeutic orientation, etc.

One factor that seems paramount (Shechtman, in Haen & Aronson, 2017) is the relationship between the child and the therapist – the therapeutic alliance. Further, she notes therapist verbal behaviors that are critical to positive outcomes. These include encouragement, interpretations and therapist self-disclosure. Another behavior that was studied was found to be negatively correlated with outcomes. This was challenging by the therapist, which was found to increase aggression and negatively impact academic achievement (p. 60). It is important to note the centrality of the relationship between therapist and child client. This emotional bond sets the stage for a therapeutic environment in the group. It is of critical importance that the therapist is aware of the transference and countertransference reactions that will shape this relationship.

Central to the interpersonal process approach to group work with children is the distinction between content and process. Two definitions from separate authors are offered.

Yalom and Leszcz's definitions:

Content: consists of the explicit words spoken, the substantive issues, the arguments advanced.

(2021, p. 185)

Process: the 'how' and the 'why' of a client's statement, especially insofar as the how and the why illuminate aspects of the client's interpersonal relationships …the meta communicational aspects of the message.

(2021, pp. 185, 186)

Smead's definitions:

> **Content:** refers to what group members are talking about, the subject of the present conversation…[content] is usually information, behavior, skills practice…that serve as a structure…
>
> (1995, p. 9)

> **Process:** refers to the nature of the relationship among the group members who are communicating with one another. Process-centered leadership focuses on the way individuals talk and what that means to the group experience.
>
> (1995, p. 10)

In the clinical vignette that follows, the content of the interaction is that children are talking about elephants at the zoo. The process elements are their struggles interacting around one member's monopolization and storytelling approach to the conversation. On a process level, much is learned about the individuals and their communication styles by focusing on the ways in which they interact. This represents very rich 'data' for the group therapist about the work to be done in the group.

Case Example: Illustration of Interpersonal Process with Children

The following vignette offers an example of interpersonal process work in the context of a children's therapy group. This vignette will offer examples of the concepts and interventions discussed in the sections that follow. The numbers in parentheses represent points that will be referenced in the subsequent sections as examples of various techniques and interventions.

This case example represents an excerpt from a therapy group for children ages 9–11. The focus of this group is on improving interpersonal skills, impulse control and developing frustration tolerance in members. The children in this group present with a number of diagnoses, but a central goal for each of the children is the development of age-appropriate self-regulatory capacity that supports healthy relationships. The group is ongoing, open-ended and meets weekly for an hour in a community mental health center setting.

The members of this group are as follows:

MATEO: A 9-year-old Latinx boy who is diagnosed with Social Anxiety Disorder. He struggles to connect with others due to his social anxiety and tends to withdraw in groups. In this session, he is more engaged and talkative. Mateo was referred by his individual therapist to develop better interpersonal skills and improved coping skills for managing his anxiety.

SALLIE: A 10-year-old White girl who is diagnosed with Disruptive Mood Dysregulation Disorder. She engages in physically and verbally aggressive behavior at home and sometimes in the community (e.g. on the playground). In other settings, she is very reserved, is frequently irritable and has a negative attitude. Sallie often appears disengaged from the group process. She was referred by her outpatient therapist to develop more age-appropriate interpersonal skills and improved coping skills for managing her anger and irritability.

PEYTON: An 11-year-old White member who is diagnosed with Oppositional Defiant Disorder. He is often verbally disrespectful, particularly toward female authority figures. He was referred by his parents in an attempt to control his escalating disrespect toward his mother. They also want him to learn better interpersonal skills with peers. Peyton comes from a family system where his father is the primary disciplinarian and his mother is more passive in response to his problem behaviors.

JEROMY: A 10-year-old Black boy who is diagnosed with Attention Deficit/Hyperactivity Disorder, Predominantly Inattentive Type. He is polite but unfocused and is quite socially adept. He likes to answer questions in the group, and will often monopolize if unchecked. He was referred by his outpatient therapist to learn better interpersonal skills and coping skills for dealing with his attention problems.

KIMMIE: A 9-year-old girl of mixed ethnicity (her mother is Chinese-American, and her father is of Native American descent). She is diagnosed with Attention Deficit Hyperactivity Disorder, Combined Type. She has poor physical boundaries with others. Kimmie often struggles to keep up with the group process due to her inattention and lack of focus. She is very energetic and enthusiastic about the group, and is its longest attending member. She was referred by her psychiatrist to learn better interpersonal skills and coping skills for dealing with her attention and impulsivity problems.

TUFAN: A 10-year-old Turkish-American boy diagnosed with Attention Deficit Hyperactivity Disorder, Combined Type. He has a very good sense of humor, but often verbalizes impulsively. This youth likes the challenge of answering questions and will monopolize at times if unchecked. He was referred to the group to address issues of focus and his tendency to draw the attention of others in the classroom through silly behavior.

This group is led by a Black male cis-gendered psychologist in his mid-50s. He is from the middle socioeconomic class and holds a Master's in Social Work degree. He is a Licensed Clinical Social Worker (LCSW) and is a native of the United States.

The group leader notices that several group members are losing their focus as Mateo talks about his day at the zoo during the initial check-in. Mateo is going into great detail about the elephant exhibit, educating the group about the difference between an African and an Asian elephant. He tends to do this quite often in the group and seems to have no awareness that he's lost his audience.

GROUP LEADER: (Noting that the other group members are not listening to Mateo) "Mateo, just a minute, I have something to ask the group…I'm noticing that the group doesn't seem to be listening to Mateo. What's going on?" (1) (3)

PEYTON: (pointing to Mateo) "That's because he's so BORING!"

GROUP LEADER: "Okay, Peyton, do you think you could find a way to say that so that it doesn't sound so negative toward Mateo? I think calling Mateo 'boring' could hurt his feelings. Is that right Mateo?" (2)

MATEO: "Yeah….(points at Peyton)…you're mean."

GROUP LEADER: "Who can help Peyton say that in a different way? Let's work on this together (4)."

JEROMY: "He could use an I-statement like we talked about last time!"

GROUP LEADER: "Okay, good idea…Peyton, do you remember how to do that?"

PEYTON: "Ummmm….no."

JEROMY: (raises his hand) "I do!"

GROUP LEADER: "Okay, Jeromy, good, but I'd like to see if Sallie can remember…Sallie, do you remember?"

SALLIE: (doesn't respond verbally, but puts her hand over her mouth)

TUFAN: "She won't talk…"

GROUP LEADER: "Well, let's give her a chance, Tufan." (5)

TUFAN: "That'll take too long!"

PEYTON: "Can you give her a chance, please, Tufan?"

SALLIE: (with her hand over her mouth) "folder."

JEROMY: "I think she said it's in her folder…can I get her folder?"

GROUP LEADER: (nods giving Jeromy permission to go to the shelf to get Sallie's group materials folder)

SALLIE: (opening her folder and pulling out the 'I-statements' worksheet from the previous week…she hands it to the Group Leader).

GROUP LEADER: "Sallie, can you read it to Peyton?"

SALLIE: (shrugs and hangs her head)

GROUP LEADER: "Would you read the first part and the group will fill in the blanks for you?"

SALLIE: (nods and begins reading from the worksheet) "I feel…"

GROUP LEADER: (to the entire group) "Good, now what feeling word can we put in, Peyton?"

PEYTON: "Bored."

GROUP LEADER: "Okay, good."

SALLIE: "When you…"

GROUP LEADER: "Okay, what caused Peyton to feel bored?"

JEROMY: "He said it was because Mateo was talking too much about the elephants."

GROUP LEADER: "Good."

SALLIE: "So, could you…"

GROUP LEADER: "…what do you want Mateo to do, Peyton?"

PEYTON: "Not go on and on about those elephants…he's, like, obsessed."

GROUP LEADER: "How can you say that in a more positive way? Does anybody have any ideas?" (6)

TUFAN: "I would just ask him to make it shorter. That would keep me from getting bored."

GROUP LEADER: "Excellent, Tufan! So, Peyton, can you borrow Sallie's I-statement sheet and read it to Mateo?"

PEYTON: (reads the I-statement to Mateo with some assistance from Jeromy and Tufan)

GROUP LEADER: "Great job, everyone. We just helped Peyton say what he wanted to say to Mateo in a way that is kind. So, what was Peyton's message to Mateo?"

JEROMY: "That he can talk about the elephants, but it shouldn't take too long or we'll get bored."

GROUP LEADER: "Mateo, is that what you heard?" (Mateo smiles and nods)

GROUP LEADER (Noticing that Kimmie's attention has drifted away from the group process): "I've noticed that sometimes it's hard for Mateo to decide how much to tell us about the things he likes. How could the group help him learn this? Kimmie, we haven't heard from you."

KIMMIE: "We could tell him in a nice way."

GROUP LEADER: "Very good. Mateo, would that be okay, if the group helps you out with that?" (Mateo smiles and nods)

Group therapists often make a distinction between interventions that are focused on individuals, subgroups or the group-as-a-whole. Yalom and Leszcz (2020) note that references to the group-as-a-whole often refer to "the group," "we" or "all of us" (p. 246). There is clearly a need for interventions focused on each of these levels. In reference to the clinical vignette above:

- Comments and interpretations at the level of the group can allow for a shift to a process focus without inducing defensiveness **(1)**.
- Well-timed comments and interventions on the individual level allow the group therapist to further the process focus **(2)**.

A process focus works to steer members away from a focus on factors outside the group and toward a focus on their relationships with one another. This facilitates learning and growth with regard to self-regulation and the ways in which one connects with others. In short, it facilitates the establishment of the interpersonal bridge discussed previously.

Smead (1995), writing about the importance of a process focus in children's groups states, "Focusing on process, on the here-and-now, helps children learn to talk about immediate thoughts and feelings, which in turn may help them in their adult relationships" (p. 10). In the clinical vignette that follows, a process approach is employed so that optimal learning and growth for members is achieved. The clinician who focuses exclusively on content might have shut down the interactions as follows, thereby missing out on the true power of group therapy:

GROUP LEADER: "OK Peyton, we don't call other group members 'boring.' That's rude and will not be tolerated in this group. Now, everybody focus and let's get on with our lesson today."

This would have missed the opportunity to engage the group in critical processing of the events as they unfold in the group. This would have denied the group valuable opportunities to learn and practice self-regulatory and self-expression strategies that support healthy relationships.

There are two stages to work in the here-and-now:

- **The activation phase**
  - ○ This involves actually shifting the focus of the group from relationships, events, etc., outside of the group to those in the group.
  - ○ In the above example, the group leader activates the here-and-now focus with the comment on the group's reaction to Mateo's storytelling **(3)**.

- **Process illumination phase**
  - ○ This involves commenting on, and thus making members aware of, interpersonal processes going on in the group.
  - ○ The clearest examples of process illumination in the above example occur when the therapist comments on what the group is currently doing or must do **(4)**.
  - ○ The combination of process activation and illumination creates what Yalom and Leszcz refer to as the *self-reflective loop* (pp. 184, 185).
  - ○ The self-reflective loop is put forth by these authors as the primary force in the interpersonal learning that occurs in group.

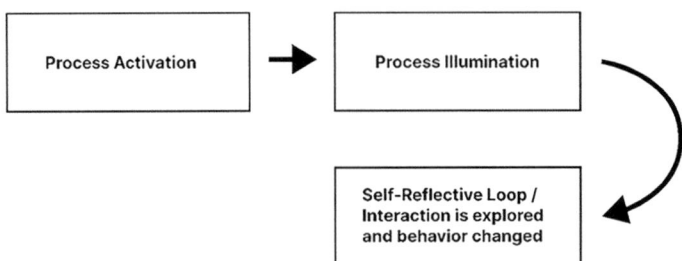

Figure 4.1 The Self-Reflective Loop Process

Process Activation

The following is another example of the self-reflective loop in a child therapy group.
- A child is prompted to practice a skill taught in the group setting (e.g., using an I-statement when appropriate).
- The child effectively uses the skill or an approximation of that skill.

Imagine an interaction between two of the members described above.
Kimmie attempts to engage Mateo in conversation during the group session.

KIMMIE: (Standing up and walking over to Mateo's chair) "Hey, Mateo are you good at math?"

MATEO: (Grunts with his lips closed) "Mmmmmm."

KIMMIE: (To the group leader) "Mr. Matt, why is Mateo acting like that? I know he can talk." (To Mateo) "Why won't you talk to me? I guess you hate me." (To the group leader) "Why does everybody hate me?"

GROUP LEADER: "I'm wondering if we can help you understand this better, Kimmie. Why don't you start by going back to your seat. I think Mateo might be a little nervous about you being so close to him. Is that right Mateo?"

MATEO: (Nods) "Yeah, you're too close Kimmie."

GROUP LEADER: "So, Kimmie it seems like when you got up to ask your question that might have made Mateo nervous."

MATEO: "Yeah, and she was too loud."

KIMMIE: "Why does everybody think I'm loud?"

GROUP LEADER: "Your question was a little loud. I know you're excited, but maybe you could try asking it sitting down and a little quieter."

KIMMIE: "OK. So Mateo, are you good at math?"

MATEO: "No. Not really. I'm better at spelling. My dad gets mad at me because I'm not good at math."

GROUP LEADER: "So you might have been a little embarrassed when Kimmie asked you that question?"

MATEO: "Yeah, a little bit."

GROUP LEADER: "Kimmie, what do you think about that?"

KIMMIE: "Well, it's OK to not be good at math. I'm not very good at spelling."

GROUP LEADER: "OK, I'd like to know what each of you learned from what we just talked about."

MATEO: "I learned that it's OK to ask somebody to sit down and ask a question more quieter if you do it nicely and that it's OK to not be good at math."

KIMMIE: "I learned that some people, like Mateo, don't like loud questions when you're standing up."

GROUP LEADER: "Great job, both of you! Those are some really important things to learn. Did anyone else in the group learn anything just now?"

The group leader responds by highlighting this process and opening up discussion with other group members who observed the interaction.

• For example: "Wow, did anyone notice what just happened with Kimmie and Mateo? What did others in the group learn?"

Despite the emphasis on a process focus, most child group therapists bring in content to their groups that is very useful. Maximizing the therapeutic benefit of group therapy involves integrating structured activities and process work. This involves the therapist continually shifting back and forth between a *content focus* and a *process focus*. The child group therapist must have a clear understanding of the objectives of the given group. These objectives will assist in decision-making regarding where the focus of intervention should be. For example, most child group therapists would agree that it is sometimes important to teach skills and provide psychoeducation. These clearly focus more on content over process. However, it is advised to be attuned to process even when engaging in more cognitively focused activities. The process focus serves to empower the learning that occurs through psychoeducation.

The following scenario provides an example of such integration:

The interaction takes place in a session focusing on making friends. The group is being led in completing an activity where they list attributes of a good friend on a worksheet containing an outline of a person. They then complete the drawing of the person (using colored pencils or crayons) with physical characteristics that represent one of their friends.

Three children become involved in an argument about who was first to write the phrase "likes the same foods that I do" on their paper. This argument begins to escalate, and it is apparent to the group therapist that none of the children will spontaneously use positive coping strategies to resolve the conflict.

The group leader intervenes drawing the group's attention away from the worksheet and to the interaction (**shifting focus from content to process**). She uses a group-as-a-whole intervention stating, "Everybody, Phillip, Annie, and Keisha are having trouble with something, let's help them out!" (**activation of the here-and-now**).

The group leader then facilitates a problem-solving session where the other children are asked to assist these three group members in resolving their conflict. Once the conflict has been resolved, the leader points out and praises the group's accomplishment (**process illumination**). This completes the self-reflective loop.

This intervention involves the use of group process that arises during a structured activity. It utilizes the in-vivo experience of the group to teach and develop positive coping skills. It employs the **social microcosm** in service of the children acquiring skills and self-awareness. The social microcosm theory (Yalom & Leszcz, 2020) states that problematic behaviors exhibited by group members outside the group will eventually emerge in the group if the process is allowed to develop. Had the therapist viewed this strictly as a discipline issue and resolved the conflict herself, the group process would have been shut down and a valuable learning opportunity for this group lost.

Bringing Discipline into the Therapeutic Milieu

Group work with children poses challenges that often don't exist in adult groups. Primary among these is management of the child's behavior in the group. An interpersonal process foundation to group work with children recasts behavior management as being a part of the group process. Such a perspective brings this aspect of children's group into the therapeutic milieu, and in doing so, greatly increases the power of the modality. There are a number of examples of this type of intervention in the previous vignette **(5) (6)**, as well as in the above scenario. Rule violations and other process issues are utilized in the group in a way that facilitates learning in the here-and-now.

Smead (1995) emphasizes the need for "ground rules" in a group and she likens these to explicit norms in groups in general. Likewise, Shechtman (2007) notes that "rules and regulations are important issues, without which chaos will characterize the group" (p. 80). Particularly with children's groups, it is often important to work together to generate these ground rules. This gives children some ownership of the group and its rules. Often, these rules are posted somewhere in the group room for reference. The following table offers a sample set of ground rules for a children's therapy group. Obviously, the specific ground rules will be determined by the needs of the given group.

Another example of setting expectations in a group is the following handout entitled "Being a Good Group Member." Such a handout can facilitate a discussion of expectations for the group.

Table 4.2 Sample Rules

Sample Ground Rules for a Children's Group

What's said in group stays in group
Hands and Feet to Yourself
One Person Speaks at a Time
Be Respectful
Use Words not Actions

Being a Good Group Member ....

- **Focus** – There's a time to be funny and a time to be serious.
  Good group members learn the difference.

- **Respect** – Everyone is in the group to learn and grow.
  Everybody is doing the best they can to be a part of the group.
  It's OK to disagree with someone, but do it with respect.

- **Listen** – Listening to each other is what makes us a group.
  Everyone will be asked to practice this challenging skill.
  It's an important part of showing respect for others.

- **Learn** – Group is a great place to practice new skills and
  learn more about yourself.

- **Share** – Good group members learn to share with each other.
  This includes sharing things in the group room (like crayons
  and paper) as well as sharing your feelings and experiences
  with others.

- **Differences** – Group helps kids (and adults) learn that it is
  OK to be different. It is very important to be able to see the
  world the way someone else sees it. There's a lot to learn
  from people who are different from you. Group brings
  different people together to learn!

Copyright 2021, Groupworks, Inc.

Figure 4.2 Being A Good Group Member Handout

Adapting the concept of the *self-reflective loop* to management of behavior will offer insight into how group process is used with children. This process involves a series of interventions that can be summarized as follows:

1   Bringing into awareness a problem faced by the group (process activation);
2   Directing and facilitating a group-level exploration (?) and problem-solving process about the problem (working in the here-and-now); and
3   Making group members aware that a problem has been identified and solved by the group (process illumination).

Such an approach can be applied to any situation where a rule violation has occurred or a conflict arises:

- Arguments over group materials (crayons, markers, etc.)
- Name-calling
- Expressions of emotions that are not adaptive (verbal or physical aggression)
- Microaggressions
- Struggles with the interpersonal resources of the group (jealousy, monopolizing, storytelling, etc.)

Working with discipline and group member behavior management in this way is presumed to work on a number of levels. *Cognitively*, there is acquisition of new skills and self-regulation capacities. Members learn methods for self-regulation through a group problem-solving approach that would not occur if behavioral problems were viewed strictly from a disciplinary perspective. On an *Interpersonal* level, children learn new ways of interacting with each other in-vivo alongside their peers. This facilitates interpersonal learning and assists with the establishment of the interpersonal bridge. On a *Neurobiological* level, we now understand that these experiences literally rewire the brain in ways that enhance self-regulation and interpersonal engagement capabilities (Siegel, 2020). Hebb's Axiom states that "neurons that fire together, wire together" suggesting that scaffolding these learning experiences changes patterns in the brain to support different ways of responding to future similar situations.

It is important to note that, in this model, the group therapist facilitates the process. Child group therapists who don't have a process focus run the risk of imposing a solution and bypassing the group process. An example of this involves the aforementioned argument over who was first to write a given item on their worksheet. Instead of facilitating a resolution with the children, the group therapist treats this as a disciplinary situation. The behavior is pointed out, and the children are given a consequence or a verbal reprimand and the content of the group is continued (worksheet, etc.). An important opportunity for learning is lost with this approach.

Behavioral Modification Techniques – Use of Reinforcements, Rewards and Consequences

Taking a process-oriented approach to managing behavior in children's groups is not exclusive of using other techniques such as behavior modification. Behavior modification techniques work well in the management of children's behavior in groups. It is neither possible nor therapeutically indicated to process every behavior or incident in a therapy group with children. As stated previously, **the goals for each group will guide the therapist in deciding what is appropriate for processing**. The use of behavior modification techniques does not entirely preclude the processing of behaviors or incidents. There are a number of **applications of behavior modification** that are useful to group leaders.

One strategy that can be useful is to withhold reinforcement for problem behaviors.

This is exemplified by a group in which one member is making inappropriate noises. These are distracting other members and disrupting the progress of the group. The group leader might have tried to process the behavior with the child, but it continues. Other group members begin to get dysregulated by this disruptive behavior. The group leader might use the following intervention:

"Everyone, Alex is trying to get our attention in a way that's not good right now. We are going to ignore that and keep on going with our activity. When Alex decides to ask for our attention in a better way, we will give it to him. Does anybody have an idea of a better way to get our attention?"

(Members brainstorm ways that Alex could gain attention more appropriately)

This approach withholds the group's attention from a member who is being disruptive. It supports the other members in learning to ignore this behavior instead of fueling it by giving the member negative attention for the behavior. It also clarifies what Alex would need to do in order to regain the group's attention in a more adaptive way. It is important to note that reinforcement of group members for ignoring the behavior is a critical point. This could be something as simple as:

"I'm noticing what a great job everyone is doing ignoring Alex's noises. I know

It can be hard to ignore, but it's important for us to do that. Great job, group!"

Another behavioral strategy is to offer a negative consequence for problem behaviors. Loss of privileges can be effective, but should be used judiciously and with compassion. Overly punitive consequences such as denial of food, overt exclusion from an activity or any other situation that might induce shame are not recommended. An example of loss of privileges that is considered appropriate is used in the following example.

The Kids Club group for elementary aged children uses a point system that is based upon children getting stamps on a weekly goal sheet (see below) for engaging in the group activities, following directions, and connecting with others in adaptive ways. These stamps are translated into points that the members can spend in the group "treasure chest," which is filled with toys and games. When members of the group engage in rule violations or behavior that is considered inappropriate, they do not receive stamps. If behavioral issues continue, stamps might be taken away. This leaves them with fewer points to spend in the treasure chest at the end of the group session.

When using negative consequences such as these, it is very important to support the child by being very clear about how they continue to earn points or prevent losing points. This should be made clear in behavioral terms. The following example provides some clarity with regard to this, using the situation with Alex from previously. The group leader might intervene in the following way:

> Alex, I noticed that you keep making noises that are distracting the group. I'd really like for you to stop doing that because you're not earning your stamps and might not have enough points to get anything from the treasure chest later. If you stop making those noises now, I can start giving you stamps again. I'd really like to be able to do that. Are you ready to stop now?

Below is an example of the aforementioned goal sheet. The reader will note that the sheet includes the child's name (in this case, Kimmie) along with their primary goal for the session. In this example, the goal is "Being More Positive." In the beginning of the session, goals are reviewed and examples of behaviors that would be consistent with the goal are solicited from each member. For example, Kimmie would be informed that her goal for the session is "Being More Positive." She would then be asked to give some examples of behaviors that would fit with this goal. This might proceed as follows:

GROUP LEADER: "Kimmie, your goal for today is "Being More Positive." Last time I think you had a hard time focusing on positive things in group. Can you give me an example of how you might be more positive today?"

KIMMIE: "Um, well, last time I got frustrated when I didn't win the game and said I was stupid and the game was stupid."

GROUP LEADER: "That's right. How could you be more positive this time?"

KIMMIE: "Well, I could say more positive things."

GROUP LEADER: "OK, we're going to play a game today. What if you lose again? How could you be more positive about it?"

KIMMIE: "I could say 'good job' to the person who wins."

GROUP LEADER: "That's a great idea, Kimmie."

As the group progresses, each member will be coached on attaining their goal. So, if Kimmie exhibits negativity, she would be gently reminded about her goal for the session. Help from other members could also be enlisted if she struggles with her goal. The grid at the bottom of the sheet is for stamps. A group member gets stamps for good behavior and for working toward their identified session goal. For example, if the group session started with a check-in on how members are doing for the week, Kimmie would get stamps or stickers for listening, paying attention and sharing.

Another example of offering negative consequences is a change in status on a progress-tracking board or level system. A simple Red/Yellow/Green level system is employed in some groups and classroom settings. A child's level can be modified depending upon how they are presenting in the group. Their level can be tied to a point system or to certain privileges. The following example demonstrates one way that this could be tied to the ability to earn prizes.

The Kids Club group for elementary school children uses a board with the designations Green, Yellow and Red. Each member has a name card that can be moved based upon their status in the group. The child's status on the board determines how many prizes they can get from the treasure chest at the end of the group. Red Status gets one small prize. Yellow Status gets two small prizes. Green Status gets three small prizes or one big prize.

In some situations, it might be necessary to use time-out for a child who cannot regulate themselves to an appropriate degree. As with some other negative consequences, this should be used sparingly, with compassion, and in a manner that does not induce shame. The following offers an example of how this might be employed using the situation with Alex from above. Alex continues to make noises in the group and it becomes so disruptive that the group leader needs to try a different intervention:

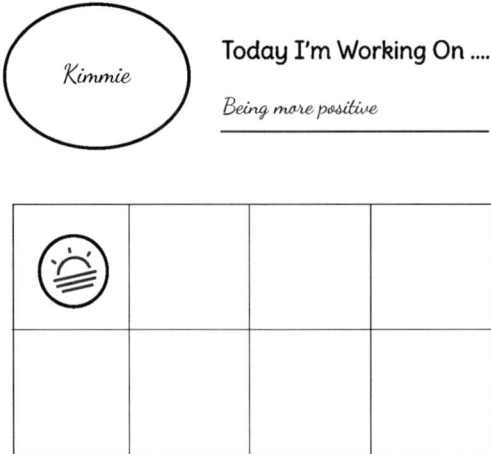

Figure 4.3 Sample Goal Sheet for Group Member

The Group Leader decides to give Alex three more chances to stop the behavior or the member will be asked to take a time-out from the group. The behavior continues, so the group leader gives another warning. Alex continues the behavior, so the group leader indicates that one more occurrence will result in a time out. Alex makes the noise another time and the group leader calmly asks the member to get up and come with them. Alex is taken to the waiting room and asked to sit with their guardian for a period of five minutes. The group leader explains to the guardian that the child is struggling with some behavior and that they need a brief time-out. The group leader sets a timer and ensures Alex that they will return to take them back to the group when the time has elapsed. At the designated time, the group leader returns and re-introduces Alex to the group.

This example assumes that the group is co-led so that someone is with the other members while one co-leader facilitates the time-out. It also assumes that a caregiver is available in the waiting room. Since neither will always be the case, modifications can be made. There could be a designated time-out space in the group room where a member could be removed from the milieu adequately but still supervised.

One of the best uses of consequences in child group therapy is employing natural consequences. A frequent natural consequence is simply disapproval from one's peers. When this is expressed, the use of here-and-now process commentary can be easily employed, as in the example at the beginning of this chapter. Another use of a natural consequence is facilitating a member apologizing appropriately for negative behavior toward someone else. The following example demonstrates the use of this. In the example, Jasmine reaches over and takes a crayon away from Hector.

The group leader notes what happened and has Hector practice using an "I-Statement" with Jasmine. Jasmine is then prompted to give the crayon back to him and to apologize. If she struggles with this, other group members can be employed to support and help her.

Another use of natural consequences involves children making something right when they act out. For example, if a child intentionally spills a drink, knocks over an item or throws items from a game; they are asked to clean up.

Thus far, consequences and rewards have been considered on an individual member level. There are also group-as-a-whole level interventions that can be effective. With this type of intervention, behavior is monitored on a group basis, and the entire group is rewarded or given a consequence. This can support group cooperation and encourage members to support each other. These types of interventions tend to work best when groups are cohesive and most members have adequate abilities to self-regulate. If there is a child or children who struggle more with this, there can be scapegoating of the member who negatively impacts the group's rewards or consequences. This will inevitably stigmatize the scapegoat who will then continue to act out after feeling bad about themselves, creating a negative loop which breaks down group cohesion. Examples of behaviors that would be rewarded on a group basis include polite reminding of peers of the group rules and working together to ensure that the group meets its goals. The following are examples of groups that might successfully employ group-as-a-whole rewards and consequences.

An anxiety management group for children includes children with good abilities in managing their behavior and anger. Most members are compliant with the group rules and respond well to group-as-a-whole rewards for practicing the skills of the group.

A highly cohesive group for children with learning differences responds well to group-as-a-whole rewards when they are on task and consequences when they get off-task. All members tend to struggle with attention and focus, so there is little potential for scapegoating that can't be managed in the context of the group.

During a group game such as bowling, teams are rewarded for being supportive of each other and using encouraging statements. If negative statements are observed, some type of penalty is applied in the game. For example, a team might lose a turn at bowling if they make negative comments toward someone.

Another example of a group-as-a-whole behavioral intervention is in the use of smiley and sad faces for desirable vs. undesirable behaviors:

A large whiteboard is used to record rewards and consequences;

A smiley face is given anytime anyone in the group engages in pro-social behavior using the 'catch them being good' principle.

Examples of behaviors that are rewarded include:

- Helping someone
- Paying attention to the group leader
- Waiting one's turn
- Sharing feelings honestly
- Practicing a skill taught in group

A sad face is given anytime anyone in the group engages in undesired behavior or a group rule violation occurs. Examples of behaviors that receive such a consequence include:

- Engaging in some behaviors without permission (leaving the room, using another member's materials, etc.)
- Speaking out of turn
- Getting out of one's seat
- Leaving or attempting to leave the group room
- Using inappropriate language
- Hitting or threatening

If one child repeatedly earns the entire group a consequence, that child is offered some 1:1 time with the group leader in order to avoid their being scapegoated based upon the repeated violations

At a designated time before the end of the session, members count their smiley and sad faces. If the smileys outnumber the sad, they each get to visit the prize box or treasure chest.

Interpersonal Considerations for Group Leadership: Ways of thinking about intervening

Without a doubt, it takes therapists with a specific set of qualities and professional abilities to work with children. Therapist and leadership style will be discussed in depth in Chapter 5, but some overlapping elements are discussed here as they directly relate to the interpersonal foundations from which groups are created.

1 **Leadership vs. facilitation** Each child group clinician will have their own leadership style. This will flow from that therapist's theoretical orientation, personality,

and professional characteristics. With regard to the interpersonal relevance of these qualities in the child group therapist, it is important to note that the child's relationship with the therapist serves a critical role in the interpersonal approach. This relationship becomes, ideally, a template for the establishment of the aforementioned interpersonal bridge. It sets the stage for the other relationships in the group. The therapist, using their personal qualities, sets the tone of the group. This, in turn, establishes an environment that is conducive to the development of self-regulatory and emotional expression capacities. This environment becomes the catalyst for the establishment of healthy and adaptive member to member relationships. Smead (1995) presents leadership style on a continuum from *leading* on one end to *facilitation* on the other (pp. 10, 11).

Leading: Therapist has complete control over the content and expectations for the session. This is similar to a classroom format where a teacher presents material in a lecture format.

Facilitation: Responsibility for what happens in the session is shared between the leader and the participants. "The group leader provides stimulus material, but the focus is on interpersonal interaction, not on learning specific content" (p. 11).While it's possible to consider where a given clinician would fall on this continuum in general, the more apt question would be where does a given clinician fall on this continuum in a given moment. Child group therapists are called upon to demonstrate flexibility along this continuum to meet the needs of their groups and the members in them. At times, leadership or a more directive, top-down approach is called for. At other times, a more facilitative approach is necessary.

Beyond leadership style, there are the basics of group leader responses to group members. Shechtman (2007) describes an investigation of six types of therapist responses in group therapy:

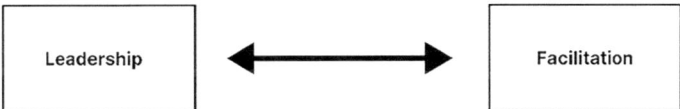

Figure 4.4 Leadership Vs. Facilitation

Table 4.3 Examples for Consideration about Leadership Approach

Leadership/Directive Approach	*Facilitative/Less Directive Approach*
There is a threat to safety in the group	The group is engaged in process-oriented work
More structured didactic material is the focus	The focus is on a less structured activity
There is a low level of self-regulatory capacity among members	There is a high level of self-regulatory capacity among members
The group, a subgroup or individuals become dysregulated	The group and its members are well-regulated

- Encourages
- Directives
- Questions
- Paraphrases
- Feedback
- Self-disclosure

Two of these leader responses, Questions and Paraphrases were found to facilitate high levels of participant self-disclosure (pp. 50, 51). Further, the use of structured activities led to greater member self-disclosure. This underscores the importance of using structured activities in groups with children alongside a process focus.

Finding the right balance between leadership and facilitation in children's groups helps to set the interpersonal tone of the group. Facilitation of the interpersonal process of the group requires the leader to make decisions about how to lead the group in a given moment. There are times when the interpersonal process demands that children's groups have strong leadership and others when gentle facilitation is more in order.

2   Kinds of interventions

Rutan et al. (2014) note three components of the therapeutic process that are important for group leaders to utilize. These components can be delivered by the group therapist or facilitated among members of the group. These are confrontation, clarification and interpretation. They are defined as follows:

Confrontation: The pointing out or identifying of some behavior or emotional state to help the group member pause and reflect on what is occurring.

An example of a confrontation by the group leader in a children's group would be for the leader to say, "Peyton, you often? talk over Sallie when she tries to speak."

These authors note that confrontations can be constructive, destructive or both (p. 95), and that "it is essential to create a supportive atmosphere that enables members to give and receive information through confrontations that are helpful and of use to other members" (p. 95).

Clarification: Refers to an elaboration or contextualizing of some behavior or emotional state. With clarification the reasons why the behavior occurs are not verbalized. This is done with interpretation.

For example, in the aforementioned example, the group leader might offer clarification by noting that Peyton seems to talk when Sallie is struggling to express herself. Other members might note that Peyton tends to talk over the girls in the group when they are talking. The group leader might add that Peyton often expresses being "bored" with the content of the group when he talks over others.

Interpretation: Involves thinking about what may be driving a particular behavior or emotional state.

In the aforementioned example, an interpretation might involve reflecting to Peyton that perhaps he talks over others when he's bored or when the pace of the group slows down. Further, an interpretation might include that he seems to feel that it's acceptable to talk over girls but not boys. The group could process this with him and help him to identify new ways of behaving that are healthier.

With each of these processes, the authors note that timing and the creation of a safe environment in which members can feel comfortable being confronted is important. It is also noted that with interpretations specifically, it is best to offer these as observations and not as "a dictum 'presented from on high'" (p. 105). There is a spirit of presenting such observations as hypotheses rather than as 'truths.'

Group Co-Leadership

Greene et al (in Kaklauskas & Greene, 2020) note that co-leadership or co-facilitation is "having more than one leader conduct a group simultaneously" (p. 133). Corey et al, (2018) note a number of advantages to a co-leadership model (p. 47):

- Group members can gain from the perspectives of two leaders
- Co-leaders can confer before and after a group to learn from each other
- Supervisors can work closely with co-leaders during their training and can provide them with feedback

Further, Rutan et al. (2014) suggest that "two therapists can more actively set limits in working with certain patient populations" (p. 223) including children and adolescents. These authors also note that the relationship between co-leaders can serve as a "model that patients can use for imitation or identification" (p. 223). With regard to cultural factors in groups, Steen, Vanmatta and Liu (in Haen and Aronson, 2017) note that having a co-facilitator who represents "different racial, ethnic or cultural backgrounds may be appropriate" (p. 261). Yalom and Leszcz (2020) write that with co-leadership, "Comparing their reactions permits a clearer discrimination between their own subjective responses and objective assessments of the interactions." (p. 62).

There are many reasons to consider a co-leadership model when working with children. Primary among these is the management of the behavior in the group itself. **Children are energetic and require oversight and behavior management in a group setting in order to ensure learning, growth and safety**. Mitchell et al. (in Haen & Aronson, 2017) note that groups addressing anger and aggression often benefit from a co-leadership model so that when "severe problem behavior" (p. 371) occurs one leader is able to work with the struggling individual while the other carries on with the group. Other populations that can benefit from a co-leadership model are those with disruptive behaviors, younger children, children who struggle with focusing and paying attention and groups that require behavioral activation such as individuals with depression.

With regard to the cons of a co-leadership model with children, there are few. Children generally benefit from the interaction between the co-leaders of the group. A co-leadership model could be detrimental to a group if the co-leaders do not have a good working relationship or if they don't share common goals for the group or a common understanding of the children in the group. It is, therefore, important that co-leaders meet often and plan group sessions together. This will ensure that their goals for the group remain aligned. Finally, group co-leaders should work through any conflict that arises in their relationships. Not doing so has potential to show up in the group and can be detrimental to the group's goals and progress.

Summary

The Interpersonal approach to groups as outlined by Yalom and Leszcz (2020) has great applicability in work with children. It is essential for the child group therapist to have an organizing model from which they work. This model permits the use of other various techniques, interventions and therapeutic models. It organizes the work of the group therapist in their interactions with child group members. Behavior modification principles allow for the management of a child's behavior in the group in a way that fosters learning and growth. The child group

---

Exercise

1   The most relevant of Yalom's therapeutic factors in children's groups appear to be: Group *Cohesiveness, Catharsis,* and *Developing Socializing Techniques.* Discuss ways to maximize the use of these in children's groups.

2   What are the two components of the *Self-Reflective Loop*? Consider ways that these components are activated and maximized by the group therapist.

3   Consider your reactions to the process focus in children's groups. How different is this from your current approach? Discuss your own foreseen challenges in implementing this approach.

4   Discuss the differences in *leading* vs. *facilitating* children's groups. Consider where you fall on this continuum. Do you need to change your style? If so, how?

5   *Behavior Modification* is used in children's groups often to manage and control actions. Discuss how integrating this with the *Self Reflective Loop* can enhance the experience of the group for children.

a   Discuss the different situations that would warrant the use of *group-as-a-whole interventions* versus *individual interventions.*

b   One example of a behavior modification system was presented in the book (offering happy or sad faces based upon behavior). Consider other such systems that you have observed, used, or that you think would be effective.

---

therapist must navigate the leadership and facilitation aspects of the group in order to align member and group goals in a way that produces change for the members of the group. The Interpersonal approach to groups can be adapted in many different forms to meet the needs of child groups!

References

Aronson, S., & Haen, C. (2017). *Handbook of child and adolescent group therapy: A Practitioner's reference.* New York: Routledge.

Corder, B. F., Whiteside, L., & Haizlip, T. M. (1981). A study of curative factors in group psychotherapy with adolescents. *International Journal of Group Psychotherapy, 31*(3), 345–354. doi:10.1080/00207284.1981.11491712

Corey, M. S., Corey, G., & Corey, C. (2018). *Groups: Process and practice.* Boston, MA: Cengage Learning.

Haen, C., & Aronson, S. (2017). *Handbook of child and adolescent group therapy: A practitioner's reference* (pp. 193–202). New York, NY: Routledge.

Kaklauskas, F. J., & Greene, L. R. (2020). *Core principles of group psychotherapy: An integrated theory, research, and Practice Training Manual.* New York: Routledge.

Kaufman, G. (1992). *Shame: The power of caring.* Rochester, VT: Schenkman Books, Inc.

Rutan, J. S., Stone, W. N., & Shay, J. J. (2014). *Psychodynamic group psychotherapy.* New York: The Guilford Press.

Shechtman, Z. (2007). *Group counseling and psychotherapy with children and adolescents: Theory, research, and Practice.* New York: Routledge.

Siegel, D. J. (2020). *The developing mind: How relationships and the brain interact to shape who we are.* New York: The Guilford Press, a division of Guilford Publications, Inc.

Smead, R. (1995). *Skills and techniques for group work with Children and adolescents.* New York: Research Press.

Yalom, I. D., & Leszcz, M. (2020). *The theory and practice of group psychotherapy.* New York: Basic Books.

5 Therapist Considerations in Groups with Children

Zachary J. Thieneman

Introduction

Therapists bring their unique attributes to clinical work. One's own cultural backgrounds, preferred clinical orientations and personality impact what the therapist does and who the therapist is. Leaders set the tone and expectations for the group as a whole – and each leader is as unique as the groups they lead!

The overlap between therapist characteristics and the therapeutic relationship in child groups is vastly complex. Many different styles of leadership can be effective across groups and clients, but no one style is consistently helpful across all groups and all clients. This chapter explores the literature of leadership styles and qualities which are likely to influence what is helpful in groups with children:

1 **Personal Qualities**: What are the personality attributes of successful child therapists which transcend theoretical orientation? How can they be applied to my child groups?
2 **Leadership Style**: Basic group leadership tasks, leadership variables which impact child groups and leader integration of different techniques and theories.
3 **Transference and Countertransference Issues**: The importance of the therapist's capacity to monitor and manage transference and countertransference to be attuned to within child groups.
4 **Use of Self in Leadership**: The impact of authenticity on therapeutic relationships and structured ways to introduce more "self" into group leadership.

The therapeutic relationship is a widely accepted factor in treatment outcome, including with children (Chiu et al., 2009). The therapeutic relationship has many different names and at its root is the fundamental concept of therapy as a relational task. The better the therapist is able to connect with children and their social systems, including families and caregivers, the better the treatment outcomes. Exploring effective leadership qualities strengthens therapy outcomes by facilitating greater relationships with a wide range of clients.

Throughout this chapter, comparisons between adult and child groups will be referenced. The reason for this is twofold: (1) all groups have a significant amount in common related to group leadership, and (2) contrasting adult and child groups highlights the requisite skills to intentionally use when working with children. Threaded throughout are regular examples from child groups used to further exemplify the distinction between the two. While reading this chapter, curiously and seriously consider your own style, personality and use of self within your child groups!

DOI: 10.4324/9781003189701-5

Personal Therapist Qualities

Therapist personality is the subject of considerable research, especially how it impacts clinical relationships. Child group therapists have many similarities to adult group therapists with a few additional, helpful qualities (Shectman, 2007). It is the work of every group therapist to connect and engage with clients. All clinicians must have a sense of goal-directed expertise to assist with their individual clients guided by both theory and personal characteristics matched to their setting.

Christiane Brems (2008) outlines positive personal qualities of successful child clinicians (pp. 6, 7):

- **Acceptance that not all children are "lovable"**; some children can easily test clinician patience and acceptance.
- **Comfort with children**. Children may act outside of expected social norms or react with intense emotions. As adult clinicians working with children, expect the unexpected!
- **Self-awareness, willingness for self-exploration and authenticity**. Awareness and exploration of self allows for better understanding of group dynamics with kids, especially as adult clinicians may respond to clients in certain ways due to personal experiences from their own childhood. Furthermore, children respond to clinicians who are authentically bringing their personality to sessions as it creates a natural predictability between the group member and the group leader.
- **Open-mindedness about values, behaviors, culture and approaches to life**. Flexibility is a key ingredient when working with children, as there are many different paths to healing.
- **Restraint from imposing own values, standards or beliefs**. Children are learning their own paths. Clinicians must work to encourage children rather than telling them how they should respond from the clinician's individual values.
- **Awareness of the impact of prejudice**. As discussed in previous chapters, prejudice has a negative impact on group interactions. Neglecting prejudice in group lessens its effects.
- **Non-offensive, non-sexist and non-racist language**. Children are often very sensitive to terms and phrases as they are tuned into the cultural happenings around them. While it may seem obvious, avoiding offensive promotes individual client values.
- **Respect for child's needs, wishes and privacy, along with accepting a child's definition of what is important**. Child groups may express certain needs which as adults we may not directly understand. However, accepting what is important to a child is accepting them and their viewpoint.
- **Awareness of child's cognitive level and limitations and adaptability to their functioning**. Discussed in length in Chapter 3, application of interventions to a child's developmental level is crucial.
- **Empathy and willingness to listen**. Children can be surprisingly long-winded and are often in places where adults do not listen. Groups provide a unique setting where the adult leader(s) adult can be empathic and excited to listen to the unique problems child clients bring into sessions.
- **Tolerance for ambiguity and tentativeness**. Children can be vague and shy during group, especially when entering a new group. Clinicians must therefore accept the tentative nature of child clients and accept vague comments during sessions.

- **Compatibility of personal style with chosen therapeutic style**. Leading child groups is not for everybody. Child clinicians must, at base, be flexible, playful, calm and compassionate. Rigidity, over-adherence to rules and emotionally charged leadership styles may be iatrogenic to the group.
- **Awareness of dress and other aspects of appearance**. Children pick up on nuances in appearance which may not seem relevant. For example, dressing up in a suit for child groups may be both impractical and set a formality to sessions which is more serious than playful.
- **Respect for and acceptance of child's caregivers**. Working with children is also working with their extended network of caregivers and parents. Respecting them and their values is an extension of the same idea with child clients.
- **Willingness to seek consultation**. There are many gray areas when working with children and having a support network of knowledgeable professionals can allow group clinicians to continue therapeutic progress even during challenging parts of group.

While this list has many relevant factors to group therapists of all ages, Brems also echoes the importance of intersectionality and development specific to child groups. **Clinician self-awareness, flexibility, confidence, creativity and respect for a child's needs/identity/culture are all key distinctions emphasized in child group work**.

Zipora Shechtman echoes the work of Brems and highlights three major personality characteristics in her seminal book Group Counseling and Psychotherapy with Children and Adolescents (2007):

- **Presence**: Enthusiasm, validation and emotional presence during the group process;
- **Self-confidence**: Risk-taking and handling resistance effectively while being open and non-judgmental and
- **Creativity**: Flexibility with group interventions which match the developmental needs of child clients while helping them to express themselves.

Corey et al. (2018) list the following personal characteristics that are important when engaging in work with children (p. 349):

- **Patience**
  - Children often challenge group leaders with unruly and oppositional behavior. An attitude of patience and understanding is essential.
- **Caring**
  - It is important for group leaders to truly care about children. Genuine connections are built upon caring.
- **Authenticity**
  - Group leaders working with children need to have an authenticity that is rooted in caring, concern and an ability to be oneself in the group room.
- **Playfulness**
  - Group leaders working with children are at their best when they can approach groups with a sense of playfulness. Play is the language of children and few characteristics are more important to clinical work with children than a strong sense of playfulness. This involves being able to make learning and interacting in the group room a fun and engaging endeavor for children. Due to the importance of playfulness as an attribute to child group leaders, it will be discussed at greater length later in this chapter.

- **A Good Sense of Humor**
  - Child group therapists must be able to laugh at themselves and the experiences of their groups. Approaching children with a joyful and humorous attitude goes a long way with regard to setting the tone of a group.
- **Ability to Tune into and Remember one's own Childhood and Adolescent Experiences**
  - It is very important for group leaders to have a sense of both the positive and negative aspects of their own experiences as youth. This is very closely tied to how the therapist monitors and manages transference and countertransference.
- **Firmness without Punitiveness**
  - There is a need to keep a group on track with its goals. While there is room for playfulness and humor, the group has work to do. Group leaders have to balance those traits with possessing enough firmness to keep the group on track. It is essential that this firmness avoid shaming and blaming of children when the need arises to set limits and boundaries.
- **Flexibility**
  - Child group therapy must be approached with a sense of flexibility. Changing plans and approaches based upon what children need is essential. While planning for groups with children is important, this must be balanced with flexibility to meet children 'where they are.'
- **Ability to Express Anger without Sarcasm**
  - Not only do many children not understand sarcasm, it is an unhealthy way to express emotion. Child group therapists should have the tools necessary to express anger in a constructive manner. This can be accomplished through modeling of I-Statements (e.g. "I feel angry when you don't do what I ask you to do. I'd like for you to do what I ask").
- **Great Concern for and Interest in Children**
  - Related to Caring and Authenticity, it is important for the child group therapist to have a genuine concern for children and an interest in their lives.
- **Optimism that Children can be Active Participants in the Healing Process**
  - It is important for the change process that the child group therapist have a core belief that children can, with the appropriate help and guidance, make improvements in their lives.

All of these overlapping characteristics encourage clinicians to think critically about client needs and how to "show up" in a way which fosters group cohesion and meets client needs.

The following example highlights the personality disposition which is uniquely important to working with children. Working with children requires the ability to "get messy," both figuratively and literally.

Imagine a scenario where clinicians and clients are working together to make "slime" as part of a broader practice of coping skills development. Think about the following two interactions:

1   Denice is finished making her slime and her hands are covered in blue and silver glitter, glue and water. She looks at the group leader, dressed in a full suit, and smiles while reaching out her hands for a 'high five.' The group leader, afraid of messing up their best suit, does not return the high five but scowls and demands Denice put her hands down until others are finished.
2   Denice is finished making her slime and her hands are covered in blue and silver glitter, glue and water. When reaching for a high five, the group leader, dressed in a full suit, returns the gesture with a high five, splattering glitter, glue and water over the area (and some on their suit). The group leader smiles and invites Denice to wait until others are finished.

If you are Denice, how would you feel in each of these interactions?

Notice the difference is not in dress, because a wide variety of professional attire is appropriate, but in the way the clinician handles the interaction. **Child therapists must be prepared to "get messy" by being flexible, open-minded, playful and aware of children's bids for connection**. Handling messiness is an excellent example of how clinician disposition and personality have the power to impact child groups.

Children are actively learning hygiene and boundaries as they develop. It is critical for child therapists to be flexible enough to handle messes and boundary crossings in a professional, non-shaming way. Adult groups rarely have to deal with sticky hands wiped on chairs, nasal mucus on a client's hand who is asking for a high five or other such occurrences commonplace in child groups. If clinicians are unable to deal with child hygiene mishaps or manage their reactions in the here-and-now of the session ("It's gross, and it will be OK" is a helpful mantra in these moments), it can negatively impact the group through inadvertent shaming. In the example above, the bid for connection from Denice could easily be missed by clinicians who are too rigid or unwilling to deal with the routine untidiness of children. Thus, clinician awareness and flexibility become important personal qualities emphasized in child group work. After all, how often does one make slime in an adult process group?

In all child groups, there are many boundary crossings which would be out of the ordinary in adult clinical work. Bromfield (2007) offers an important overview of the clinical boundary exceptions commonplace in work with children. Child therapists must use their judgment about things like snacks, physical affection, gift-giving and other boundaries. Bromfield states:

> …we must build our therapies on strong and dependable frameworks. Indeed, we can't afford to do otherwise. Ignoring the framework will nearly always lead to erratic, unreliable, and weak–if not abusive or dangerous–therapy experiences. Embracing it too rigidly, however, without room for the necessary adaptations to the child's fluctuating needs, will forsake some of the golden opportunities for therapeutic intervention and growth. We must remind ourselves that there are no absolute right or wrong answers. The right answers we seek are much more complex, variable, and changeable.
>
> (p. 157)

Just like child groups have messes, activities and play, they also might include snacks, drinks or fist bumps and high fives. In groups with children, these moments are critical. If a child group leader is overly rigid, then the child might feel shame or guilt over what is a normal connective moment elsewhere in their life. If a child group leader is overly diffuse with boundaries, then they might do a disservice to the client by inadvertently refusing to talk openly about their actions. Clinical judgment is key. One important question to ask, which can be done in so many variations, is: "What's the function: that is, what is the meaning of this event and what does it serve for those involved?" Why does this specific child want to bring me a gift? Why do they seek a hug after each session? Why do they want to know specific things about my personal life? Asking yourself the function – the motivations and intentions – of a certain behavior can also bring it into the here-and-now processing of the group session. The following clinical vignette illustrates this point.

An outpatient group led by two clinicians meets at a community mental health center twice a week. There are seven children ages six to eight. One particular member, Elle, is always waiting at the entry room to immediately hug the clinician, regardless of who opened the door. The same dynamic is apparent with the other members in the group (as well as at Elle's school, church, and even strangers), as she often gives them hugs spontaneously.

The co-leaders expressed curiosity about the ambush hugging and consulted about it following group one night. They decided to ask the question "What's the function?" and explore it during the next session.

It happened at the beginning of the session as usual. One of the leaders opened the door to the group room and was immediately given an unexpected hug. Upon entering the group room, Elle then gave a hug to another member while expressing excitement for sitting next to her "bestie." Before the leaders could say anything, another member asked: "Why do you give everybody hugs all the time?" Elle paused for a moment and answered: "I want you to feel loved." The group leaders shared a moment of eye contact, realizing the importance of Elle's hugging. One of them followed up: "You know, I want you to feel loved, too. I have two thoughts. One, I wonder if there are times you do not feel loved? I would like to hear about them if so. Two, sometimes people like their personal space. I bet you can help people feel loved without hugging them by surprise. Our bodies have boundaries and we need to ask consent before touching another person. Would that be okay?"

Following this interaction, the group talked about boundaries, affection and expressions of care. Elle then began to ask for permission with physical affection and started expressing her care verbally. As a result, her interpersonal relationships inside and outside of group blossomed. She developed several close friends at school and really did find a "bestie" in the group itself. All of this stemmed from a curiosity about Elle's actions, how they related to her feelings and how they present in group sessions.

The clinicians in this vignette could be overly rigid (rejecting the display of affection entirely or even rudely) or diffuse with their boundaries (allowing the hugs to continue without addressing them). Neither would be in Elle's best interest. Situations like this are common in child group work and are an important distinction from work with adults. **Every child therapist must carefully consider the emotional and behavioral function of boundary crossings and how they relate to client needs**. This requires significant clinician awareness and flexibility which are vital to success with child groups.

Playfulness and Humor

Children learn through play. Too often, even in kid-focused settings such as schools, children are demanded to sit still and passively receive information. Lectures, long periods of sitting and reading or hours-long testing protocols are simply not suited for children. This goes against the natural inclination of children to explore, be active and *learn by doing*. Clinicians working with kids may often forget the importance of play amidst the seriousness therapeutic work brings. As a child clinician, sometimes we simply need to stop, breathe and remember the perspectives of our child clients. If we put ourselves in their shoes, we remember the importance of play and humor. A playful, humorous, fun adult teaching emotional regulation skills makes the learning less "classroom" and considerably more engaging and as such, *more likely for children to understand and practice the skills*. Group therapy offers the opportunity for activity-focused therapeutic endeavors which 'play' to children's strengths.

Imagine the following group of children who are in an intensive outpatient (IOP) setting where they spend upwards of two-hour blocks in group therapy once a day. This particular IOP at a specialty clinic is for children on the autism spectrum disorder (ASD). The group has been together for roughly two weeks and are in a prominent working phase. During the group session, the focus is learning social rules regarding seriousness and playfulness. More specifically, the group is learning appropriate times to be silly, appropriate times to be serious and how to read the emotional tones of others in the group before socially engaging.

- **Jeremiah** is an 11-year-old white, cisgender male diagnosed with autism, level one without intellectual or language impairment. He has a long history of treatment interventions starting with applied behavioral analysis starting when he was five when he was diagnosed with ASD. He was referred for a rigid playstyle and not knowing how to engage peers.

- **Nico** is a 13-year-old Korean-American, cisgender male adopted into a white family. He is diagnosed with autism, level one without intellectual or language impairment. He was diagnosed when he was ten after struggling to make friends in school. He highly prefers animals and collects them at home, but pets and wild animals such as frogs and caterpillars.
- **Tina** is a 10-year-old white, cisgender female. She is diagnosed with autism, level two, without intellectual or language impairment. Tina was diagnosed at a young age and is considered a savant due to her high intelligence and eidetic memory. Tina often gets into trouble at school for physically pushing away peers and prefers to spend her time alone.
- **Trey** is an 11-year-old biracial (mother is white, father is Chinese), cisgender male diagnosed with autism, level two, without intellectual or language impairment. Trey is highly social and enjoys spending time with his friends but needs frequent breaks from them. When in social situations for too long or during times he is requested to be flexible, he may verbally lash out at peers or attempt to control their choices while playing.
- **Adam** is a 10-year-old biracial (mother is black, father is white), cisgender male. Adam is diagnosed with autism, level one, without intellectual or language impairment. He is the newest to the group and was diagnosed at the clinic due to a referral from school where he experiences social rejection and emotional outbursts when unexpected changes, such as the loss of a game, occur.
- Group leader one is a biracial, transmasculine therapist from a high socioeconomic status and master's degree in marriage and family therapy. He is native to the United States.
- Group leader two is a White, cisgender female from a middle socioeconomic status with a master's degree in clinical social work. She is native to the United States.

GROUP LEADER ONE: "Hello everybody! How are you today?"

ADAM: "Good."

TREY: "I'm super good, my mom is taking me to get tacos after this. Tacos are my favorite. They are crunchy and I could eat a million of them."

NICO: "I can't believe you eat those. They're the worst."

TREY: "No they're not-"

GROUP LEADER TWO: "Trey and Nico, it's okay to think differently about tacos. Remember, we focus on flexibility and growth mindset- not 'rock brain'!"

NICO: "Okay. I'm just saying, tacos, especially fast food tacos, are gross."

GROUP LEADER TWO: "Your opinion is always valid and heard. How are you, Nico?"

NICO: "Good."

GROUP LEADER TWO: "Cool. How about you, Tina and Jeremiah?"

JEREMIAH: "I am doing well. Thank you for asking. And how have you been these past 24 hours since our last meeting?"

GROUP LEADER TWO: "You are kind to ask, Jeremiah. I am doing great, but probably not as great as Trey because I am not eating tacos after group."

JEREMIAH: "So you would be better with tacos? You should go with Trey."

GROUP LEADER TWO: "Maybe I should, though maybe I shouldn't. Tacos taste good to me but my body doesn't like them for too long. Tina, how about you?"

TINA (doesn't respond): "…"

GROUP LEADER TWO: "Tina- hey! Can I get your attention so I know you're listening? (Tina looks up) Thank you- how are you today?"

TINA: "Good. I was just watching Alice in Wonderland in my head. The queen of hearts is scary."

GROUP LEADER TWO: "That's a great movie. While you're in group today, would you mind trying to focus on what we are doing? Movies are pretty awesome, but I like group better when you're here with us. Can you do that for us today?"

TINA (thinking for a moment): "I hit pause."

GROUP LEADER TWO: "Thanks. Alright, are you going to introduce our goals for the day?"

GROUP LEADER ONE: "Sure thing. Today, we are all going to be practicing the same thing: knowing when to be serious and when to be silly. Do you know what I mean? (heads nod yes) Okay, great. Nico, can you tell me what I mean by being serious vs. silly?"

NICO: "No."

GROUP LEADER ONE: "Alright then. Adam, what about you?"

ADAM: "I don't know what you mean."

GROUP LEADER ONE: "Hold on a second. Does anybody actually know what I mean? (group nods no, group leader smiles and laughs) Well, you could have just said that at the beginning. It's always okay to not understand something. We are here to learn! What does it mean to be serious?"

TINA: "Wednesday Addams."

ADAM: "What about me? It's Thursday."

GROUP LEADER TWO: "I think she means the movie character. Addams family, right?"

TINA (nods): "Yes. Wednesday Addams is very serious. She doesn't smile or laugh a lot. She just walks around like this." (Tina stands up and walks around, looking solemn with her hands at her side)

GROUP LEADER ONE: "That's a surprisingly nice comparison, Tina. Good work! Have you all seen the Addams Family? (some nods yes, some no) Check it out sometime, friends. Like Wednesday Addams, being serious means focusing your attention, being kind, not laughing, and showing others you are listening. People might be serious when they are concentrating on a test, sitting in prayer with their family, listening to a friend having a bad day or when playing a sport. I would guess that most of you know what it means to be silly? (group nods) I've noticed in group that sometimes when we are talking about a serious topic, somebody makes a joke which ends up being upsetting rather than funny. I have also seen some of you try and talk about something serious when the group is laughing. Knowing when to be serious or silly involves you as the group members paying attention to the emotions of the other people and what we are talking about before you speak up. You have funny jokes and I want to hear them, just not when somebody is talking about fighting with their parents. You all matter and I want you to feel listened to when you are talking in our group. This skill will help that!"

GROUP LEADER TWO: "I think so, too. You each have important things to say. In group, we practice listening to each other just like you would want people to listen to you. Say, do you have any jokes?" (looking at group leader one)

GROUP LEADER ONE: "I do! What's an astronaut's favorite part of a keyboard? The space bar! Ha!"

GROUP LEADER TWO: "Wow, that was funny! I have a joke, too: I hate it when people say age is just a number. Age is clearly a word."

GROUP LEADER ONE (laughing): "Great joke! Okay, so we are going to move back and forth between two different activities: talking about our week and playing Uno. I have a very special switch here. You see when the switch is flicked "on" it points to serious. When the switch is "off" it points to silly.

ADAM: "Switches are for lights."

GROUP LEADER ONE: "They often are. This switch is special. I made it just for being serious and silly. It doesn't work on the lights, though. So when we are practicing being serious, I want people to remember Tina's example of Wednesday Addams and use your listening bodies so that whoever is talking knows you are listening. When we are practicing being silly, I want you to practice being silly while also being respectful. This means you might practice telling a joke when it's your turn during Uno or you might talk about something funny that happened during school. Do you understand? (group nods yes, therapist squints eyes) …okay, I'm trusting you on this one."

GROUP LEADER TWO: "Let's start with Uno. Note that our switch says serious. How many of you have played Uno before? I know Jeremiah and Adam really wanted to play Uno yesterday. (each member raises their hand) Great. Let's play Uno while we check in about our day."

(Group focuses intently on playing Uno. Around ten minutes later…)

GROUP LEADER TWO: "Wow, you have been SERIOUS about Uno. I am giving everybody a few extra stickers for doing so well being serious."

GROUP LEADER ONE: "That's fantastic. I think it's time to flip the switch to silly. Let's keep playing Uno and talking!" (flips fake switch to silly)

(A few minutes go by but nothing changes) GROUP LEADER TWO: "I don't know about you, but I don't feel like anybody is really practicing being silly."

GROUP LEADER ONE: "I agree. Anybody know any jokes? There are lots of ways to be silly, but we might need to break the ice a little bit."

JEREMIAH: "Marcus told me one."

TREY: "Who's Marcus?"

JEREMIAH: "My behavior therapist. He told me one joke I need to remember."

GROUP LEADER: "What's the joke?"

JEREMIAH: "What's blue and not very heavy?"

TREY: "…what?"

JEREMIAH: "Light blue."

GROUP LEADER TWO (laughing): "That's hilarious! I'm giving you an extra check for being brave and telling your joke. How did it feel to tell your joke?"

JEREMIAH: "Good. I felt good when we all laughed."

TREY: "You should, because that is the funniest joke EVER. I have a joke, too. What do you call a person who never farts in public?"

NICO: "…Well, what?"

TREY: "A private tutor!"

(Group begins laughing)

GROUP LEADER ONE: "I love your jokes! You're doing such a good job being silly. Trey, I am also giving you a sticker for being brave and telling a joke, even if it was about farts. You all have been doing so great with Uno. I would also like to hear about your days, so why don't we pause for just a few minutes. How have you all been feeling today? Does anybody have a high or low they would like to start with?"

ADAM (suddenly standing up): "I was NOT FINISHED playing Uno! I am done with this group. It's stupid."

GROUP LEADER TWO: "I can see you are feeling angry about switching from playing Uno to talking about our day. It's always okay to feel. Just remember that when things aren't going our way, the best we can do is to go with the flow like a cooked spaghetti noodle. If you need a break, you can have one. Just remember you will only earn checks when you participate in the group." (Adam looks ahead and does not respond)

GROUP LEADER ONE: "Nico, can you tell us about your day? We are being silly here, so feel free to tell us something funny that happened."

NICO: "My mom and I were driving yesterday and we saw a dog!" (Nico pauses)

GROUP LEADER ONE: "…tell us more. Was the dog doing something?"

NICO: "Yeah, it had its head out of the window like with its tongue out like this." (Nico imitates sticking his head out of a window and putting his tongue out with wide eyes, to which the group laughs)

TREY: "Are you sure it wasn't like THIS?" (Trey imitates Nico but more exaggerated)

NICO: "Yes! You're hilarious!"

ADAM (laughing and smiling): "Was it a dog sticking his head out of the window or was it you?" (Nico pretends to stick his head out of the window while he and Adam laugh)

GROUP LEADER TWO: "Welcome back, Adam. I am glad you are willing to participate again. I'm going to give you a sticker for working hard to rejoin the group. I also liked that you were paying attention to how the group was laughing and being silly. That was a good time to make a joke!"

GROUP LEADER ONE: "Nico, I like your story. Alright, let's take a moment to relax because I am going to flip our switch back to serious. Remember, being serious means we are focusing, paying attention and practicing kindness while listening or speaking. Does anybody have anything serious they would like to bring up?"

ADAM (raising his hand): "I do. A friend of mine, well, I guess we aren't friends anymore but we used to be, we used to play games together online. We were playing Fortnite and I beat him in a round and he called me a Mudblood."

JEREMIAH: "What's Mudblood mean?"

TINA: "It means 'dirty blood.' Mudblood's a foul name for someone who's Muggle-born. Someone with non-magic parents. Someone like me. It's not a term one usually hears in civilized conversation."

GROUP LEADER ONE: "From Harry Potter, yes. For those who do not know about Harry Potter, what does that mean?"

TINA: "I guess he was making fun of you for your blood, I think. When Draco Malfoy called Hermione a Mudblood, he was being a bully. Whoever you were playing with on Fortnite is not your friend. "

GROUP LEADER TWO: "Tina you're saying Adam's online friend was trying to be a bully? (Tina nods) I agree, it sounds like he was trying to be mean. Adam, how are you feeling about the situation?"

ADAM: "Bad. I thought he was my friend. I guess not anymore. It's not the first time somebody has made fun of me. They usually make fun of me for my skin."

TREY: "People make fun of me for my skin all the time. It feels… really bad."

NICO: "Me too! Some kid said that to me last week. They say I should go back to where I came from. But I came from here, just like them. I grew up here."

GROUP LEADER ONE: "I appreciate each of you sharing. I can relate to those experiences, as people have told me to go back to where I came from. Or told me I don't belong somewhere, sometimes even in bathrooms. It hurts. Sort of like a sting to my feelings which hurts more every time it happens. Is that how you all feel?"

(Nico, Trey, and Adam all nod)

GROUP LEADER ONE: "Adam, how do you feel about it?"

ADAM: "I feel bad, sort of like they were my friend but now they're not. Trash. I feel like they are throwing me away."

NICO: "You're not trash! You're my friend!"

TREY: "Yeah! You're the best. We can play Fortnite together."

GROUP LEADER TWO: "Wow, it sounds like you all really want Adam to feel different. How do you want him to feel?"

NICO: "Good. The best."

TREY: "Not like trash, that's for sure." (Adam smiles)

ADAM: "Thank you. I'm not trash because I don't stink." (Adam laughs and Nico and Trey start laughing)

GROUP LEADER TWO: "That's very kind of you all. Thank you for being brave enough to bring this up. I can't know what it's like to be you. I do know what it is like for people to be cruel based on who you are or what you look like. I am going to give Adam, Trey and Nico an extra sticker for working so hard to communicate your experiences. (Nico, Trey and Adam smile confidently) You belong here, just as you are. I also want to point out how the group was really respectful while we were talking about a serious topic. Thank you. Adam, how do you feel? You got some really great support from Nico and Trey."

ADAM: "Good. I like having friends in here. I can be me in group."

GROUP LEADER ONE: "That's wonderful, Adam. We want you to be you – exactly as you are – and know that you are great. I'm going to give the whole group an extra sticker for paying attention to the emotions of the room and staying serious. Would it be okay to switch back to silly? You all have worked so hard during our serious time. (Group nods) Okay, let's also go back to Uno. Nico, can you do us a favor and pretend to be the dog hanging out the window to help us get back into silly mode?"

Think about the ways in which humor and playfulness were used in the above vignette. Taking the time to process member interactions allowed for humor and authenticity while group leaders flexibly modeled how to be serious when necessary. The group leaders often played off each other to make jokes and prompted the group to practice in-vivo social skills about seriousness and silliness. In this vignette, the group was able to fundamentally use levity as a way to further the group's work. The example above weaves in content and process to show the multilayered ways group leaders can set the tone for groups. Notice that in this scenario, the group leaders took the emotional leads of the clients and even used self-disclosure as a way to create an emotional connection with members. During times of silliness, leaders made verbal and non-verbal communication to be silly. During times of seriousness, leaders modeled how to talk about feelings in an open, vulnerable and non-judgmental fashion. The shared emotions and experiences ultimately helped Adam feel differently. Nico and Trey's validating support was clearly impactful to Adam. The vulnerability, emotional expression and support from the group members were reinforced by group leaders.

Reflecting back on the group, if you were the leader, how could you have used humor or playfulness in a different way which reflects your own style? If you were the therapist, how would you have handled the situation Adam brought up?

Concluding Thoughts on Leader Characteristics

Infusion of effective child leadership personality characteristics can greatly change group dynamics in a positive way. Many personality styles are capable of successful leadership with child groups. The clinician characteristics above may come more or less naturally to any given clinician. If one or more are absent or challenging for an individual leader, it does not preclude positive outcomes. However, general characteristics such as playfulness, flexibility, compassion and respect for diversity provide helpful ideas of how to lead groups in an encouraging, affirming manner and are worth integrating. An attitude of enthusiasm, for example, may easily be integrated when greeting children at the start of a therapy session regardless of therapist mood or interpersonal style.

In short, our ability to create a warm, flexible and compassionate environment for our child clients is an especially important task for children who enter into therapy often feeling rejected, neglected, or dysregulated. **The therapeutic environment starts with you as the group leader knowing what your strengths, weaknesses and overall personality bring to the group room**. The more you know yourself, the better you are equipped to handle the range of diverse clients which walk into your office. Our own modeling sets up a healing environment which starts with the way we present during group sessions.

Leadership Style

Therapeutic style is closely tied to clinician preference, orientation and client needs. Leadership style is highly dependent on the individual group, leader personality and the context in which the group occurs. For example, outpatient process groups are starkly contrasted by in-patient psychoeducational groups or long-term residential therapy groups and as such dictate different styles to meet the demands of the system.

Leadership style may be defined as the ways in which group leader(s) choose to engage with, deliver and respond to group content, the group as a whole, its members and interactions between them. This includes therapist disposition (as discussed above in therapist personality), general tasks during group and the processes through which leaders create change. In discussing leadership style, it remains imperative to critically consider one's therapeutic leadership style to develop more conscious intentionality of interventions and how they are delivered.

Group leaders, regardless of the population or age of the group, are set with specific tasks. Rutan et al. (2019) in Kaklauskas and Greene's Core Principles of Group Psychotherapy describe the **basic tasks of group leadership including shaping norms, setting and maintaining time and other boundaries, creating safety, fostering therapeutic engagement, establishing individual therapeutic alliances with members and establishing therapeutic alliance with the group as a whole**.

Regardless of style, basic tasks are the work of every group. They are integral to the development of any group and are established through leader *consistency*, *reliability* and *dependability*. Regardless of therapeutic orientation or setting, such characteristics form a sense of security and predictability which set the stage for therapeutic change in child groups. Style, therefore, stems from how basic tasks are established, enforced and maintained over the course of group.

Leadership style can be correlated to the process of a group, the how specific actions occur within a group itself. All group leaders have their own ways in which they respond to displays of emotions, conflict between group members, psychoeducation moments and other therapeutic tasks. Clinicians often use therapy terms such as validation, open-ended questions, reflections, encouragement, limit setting and feedback to describe their own responses to clients. This is the heart of leadership style – how clinicians choose to respond to their specific child groups based on complex group-, client- and clinician-specific factors. Developing a sense of intentionality through leadership style allows more choice and expertise for the child group leader.

As discussed in Chapter 4, Smead (1995) offers a useful **continuum between leadership and facilitation**. **Leadership**, on one end, is more of a classroom-style control of a group direction while **facilitation** is non-directive, focusing on the leader providing stimulus material but the learning itself is derived from the interpersonal dynamics between members. Most group leaders employ a mixture of both styles, as working with children also requires a level of "crowd control" in order to engage in any therapeutic work. **Thus, more often with younger children, groups (even process-oriented groups) are often more directive and "leadership" oriented than groups with teens or adults**.

Beyond basic therapeutic tasks, leadership style also influences process and outcomes. Leaders set the tone and act as models for group members to follow. For example, Shectman and Toren (2009) found that meaning attribution and support impact both process and outcomes while stimulation, use of self, and other process variables impact interpersonal relationships reported by group members.

Despite being a vastly complex subject, Shechtman and Toren's research points to how leadership style impacts broader group outcomes. Group leadership impacts members' abilities to engage with others inside and outside of the group. In child groups, leaders model how to express feelings and respond adaptively to others. Leadership style dictates how the individual leader models positive social communication. Both easy to see and difficult to pinpoint, leadership greatly impacts child group functioning.

Leadership style, like personality in group leadership, has significant overlap between adult and child groups. However, key differences remain which uniquely impact child groups. **Shechtman (2007) discussed six types of therapeutic responses for child groups**:

- Self-disclosure (talking about one's self in relation to client experiences)
- Feedback (providing specific information about client behavior)
- Encouragement (promoting specific behaviors or engagement)
- Directives (instructing clients to take specific actions)
- Questions (asking…)
- Paraphrases (summarizing group or client experiences)

In this same work, Shechtman found **structured activities** and **questions** resulted in 90% of client self-disclosure. After all, children require developmentally-targeted activities to grasp therapeutic concepts and foster group cohesion. Shechtman's work serves as a healthy reminder of therapeutic intentionality with child interventions.

Child group therapists are often more active, directive and engaging than in adult groups. Most adult group leaders are familiar with paraphrases, questions and feedback which are commonplace in adult groups. However, self-disclosure, encouragement and directives are more common in child groups than in adult groups.

Think about a group member who is making jokes while in a group talking about sadness, disrupting other members. Imagine the following brief responses:

- "I am feeling frustrated with your jokes while we are talking about sadness. (Self-disclosure)
- "You are distracting other members when you make jokes." (Feedback)
- "I have seen you be serious before when talking about feelings, I know you can today!" (Encouragement)
- "I would like you to stop joking while we talk about sadness." (Directive)
- "It seems like you are having a hard time talking about sadness. Can you tell me what's going on?" (Question)
- "You are telling jokes while we talk about sadness." (Paraphrase)

While simple examples, these responses provide a window into how child group process differs from adult process through leadership style. In order to effectively manage child groups, different strategies are employed such as directives, encouragement and self-disclosure. The emphasis on style includes clinician-specific preferences. Child group leaders tend to be more directive and straight-forward because of childhood development. Using advanced figurative, abstract language simply isn't effective in child groups. The here-and-now processing in child groups is concrete and to the point.

Leadership style incorporating Shechtman's therapeutic responses are developmentally sensitive ways to "speak child" with clients who need more direct language and limit setting during group sessions. In an interpersonal dance, children "pull" for more straight-forward responses.

Children are curious and often ask personal questions, leading to increased self-disclosure. Child clients might ask about the clinician's children; they routinely ask about the same preferences or experiences they are sharing during the group; and in a co-leader model, children are likely to ask if the clinicians are partnered. Frequently, children will ask you about your favorites, usually within the context of their preferred topics. While you might not have a favorite rescue vehicle, some children do and want to know yours. While all of these could come up during adult groups, children are far more likely to ask personal questions without context. Child group leaders, therefore, must have established ways to handle direct questions which might seem abrasive or intrusive for the adult clinician. The motivation behind children's inquiries is starkly contrasted from that of adults. While some adults may seek personal therapist information for ulterior motives, children largely seek it out of plain curiosity. Self-disclosure then becomes a way to connect with children rather than a boundary-crossing, though clinical discretion remains crucial during any time of self-disclosure. **The interpersonal dynamics stemming from the bold curiosity of children lead to nuanced differences which distinguish adult and child groups**.

Exercise

Think for a moment about your general leadership style. Do you tend to be more directive or passive? What kind of techniques are you uncomfortable employing? How do you often choose to respond to your child clients during group/what is your "modus operandi" when interacting with child groups? Compare and contrast your leadership style with that of a trusted colleague or mentor. How are they different? How are they the same? In what ways would you like to be more intentional with your group leadership?

Transference and Countertransference

The concepts of transference and countertransference are deeply steeped in the history of psychodynamic psychotherapy. From a relational standpoint, it is easy to see why. Child clients frequently experience clinicians in the familiar ways they have come to experience parental or caretaking authority figures in their lives. **Just like the developing child mind projects personal experiences onto play scenarios, children transfer relational feelings onto therapists**.

Many modern branches of psychotherapy use the notions of transference and projective identification as a way to provide a window into the lives of clients (Lini & Bertrando, 2020). Altman et al. offer a thorough review of influential transference and countertransference history in *Relational Child Psychotherapy* (2002). Some of the pioneering researchers of child relational therapy including Melanie Klein, Anna Freud and Donald Winnicott theorized many of the basic tenants for effective child therapy *still used today.*

As theorized by Klein, A Freud and Winnicott, children readily project onto the immediate situation - including the therapy group- their feelings, perceptions and attitudes towards internalized images of parents and other caretakers, thus allowing the clinician to come to understand what underlying emotional and relational needs are driving disruptive behaviors and problematic relationships in the here and now of the therapy group. The group becomes a holding environment for therapeutic change where clinicians can help meet client emotional and relational needs.

These dynamic concepts remain relevant in standards of care for child therapy and are particularly meaningful within child groups. It is useful to understand the play activities and interpersonal dynamics that arise within the therapy group as projections of the child's internal world onto the actual here-and-now participants in the group. Sometimes leaders are seen as parental figures, teachers or family members while other members may be seen as siblings, friends, or bullies. Whatever the unique transference dynamics, group therapists must monitor and manage multiple transferential relationships and reactions while managing their own countertransference reactions effectively (Wanlass et al., 2006). Yalom and Leszcz write: **"transference is so powerful and so ubiquitous that the dictum 'the leader shall have no favorites' seems to be essential for the stability of every working group"** (2020, p. 262). The externalized emotional and relational dynamics (examples in parentheses) that constitute transference take many forms with children such as:

- Opposition to authority ("I'm not going to do what you want me to do")
- Fearful Reactions to others based upon traumatic experiences of abuse or neglect ("I do not like you or what you said to me")
- Distrust ("I do not trust you or the group")
- Need for control ("I want to play this game, now")
- Resistance to structure and rules ("I don't like talking about feelings")
- Patterned ways of eliciting needed attention from others ("I need you to laugh at my joke")
- Monopolizing ("I need you to listen to me, now")
- Crying ("I have emotions which need to be seen")
- Withdrawing ("No thank you, I refuse to participate")
- Making demands ("If we don't play my game, I'm leaving")
- Reacting differentially to group leaders based upon the leader's gender identity ("You're not my mommy, I don't have to listen to you")

No matter how transference shows up within groups, it must be dealt with through interpersonal processes so children may develop new, adaptive resolutions. When considering transference with children, the phenomenon of transference likely involves more present-oriented relational dynamics. Children simply have less relational history than adults. Since they also have less relational history in general, they are more likely to superimpose feelings and understandings from their families of origin onto present situations. In other words, children are primed to interact with others based upon their immediate family experiences.

Regardless of the way in which transference manifests itself in the group, it must be identified, explored, interpreted, then provided with a corrective experience in the context of interpersonal group processes for change to occur. Despite the behavioral manifestation of transference, the goal is to guide the child in resolving the situation in new and more adaptive ways. Factors such as culture, ethnicity and other factors in the family will influence that child's experience of others, and therefore, their transferences. It is important for the child group therapist to consider how transferences might vary based upon the intersecting identities of the child and their family.

Imagine a group scenario specifically related to Zion, an eight-year-old cisgender middle boy of four siblings whose mother died in an auto accident a year prior, leaving his father as a single parent. Zion's father appears significantly stretched thin between work and family responsibilities, either bringing him late or having another family member bring him. Zion frequently struggles with emotional regulation, trauma reactions, and overall feelings of being left out and behind. Zion is having a transference reaction to the group as a whole, recapitulating his family experience:

GROUP LEADER: "We have two games to choose from today, Hot Bomb-Ball (a fictional "Hot Potato" style game) and Statue City (a freeze tag-inspired game). Can everybody please close their eyes for just a moment so we can secretly choose a game together?"

(The group chooses Statue City)

ZION (emotionally upset, begins to yell): "I NEVER get to choose the game! It's always what YOU want, or what HE wants, or what SHE wants (pointing to other members)! IT'S NEVER WHAT I WANT!" (At this point Zion starts to cry and hit his chair)

GROUP LEADER: (Grabs the remote control to "Pause" the rest of the group) "Friends, would you mind if we paused for a second? We have somebody who is upset and we care about him. Zion, I can see you are angry and maybe sad. Would you like to talk about it now or wait a minute to calm down?"

ZION: (Nods with force)

GROUP LEADER: "So what is your choice?"

ZION: (slowly starting to stop crying while refusing to look at the group leader) "…talk."

GROUP LEADER: "Thank you for making a choice, I am always happy when we are able to talk about our feelings. Can you tell me about what you are feeling?"

ZION: "I am SO ANGRY (Zion starts to increase in volume and action) that we NEVER get to play MY games!"

GROUP LEADER: "I can see that you are angry. Would you be able to talk in a lower volume with me? I want other friends here to feel safe and sometimes yelling doesn't feel safe. Would it be okay if we just sat and waited for a moment? We are here with you when you are ready."

ZION: "Ok… (Still crying softly, after about a minute begins to talk) I never get to choose at home. It's always THEIR turn. My dad never notices, he's always busy. Or tired. Or not around. I just want it to be MY turn. It was ALWAYS my turn with my mom."

GROUP LEADER: "It sounds like you feel left out, especially at home, and that you miss your mom. It sounds painful and sad to remember your mom while always doing what your siblings want to do. Here in group, we practice things a little differently. That's part of what makes group so special. Do you feel like we listen to you?"

ZION: (nods)

GROUP LEADER: "Good. We care about you and want you to feel heard and seen. Maybe we can find a way so we all get to take turns and choose our game? How would that feel for everybody?"

(Cheers from the group, including Zion who smiles as he wipes his eye)

GROUP LEADER: "Friends in group, you have been so patient listening to me and Zion. How can we take turns choosing our games?"

CINDY: (somebody Zion really admires and gets along with raises her hand) "Zion, you're like, one of the coolest people I know. You're always so brave and nice. You're basically my best friend. Can Zion choose the game today?"

GROUP LEADER: "I appreciate your kindness to Zion. Zion, did you hear how much Cindy admires you? (Zion nods) We voted on a game for today, but I am wondering if we can choose a new way to pick games for the next time. Cindy, do you have any ideas?"

CINDY: "…can Zion pick next time? I want him to choose."

GROUP LEADER: "Yes, that's possible. How would you all feel about taking turns each week so that everybody can choose the game they want to play? (The group nods) Great! Do you all agree to play the game somebody else wants, even if it's not the game you want to play that day? (The group nods again) Excellent. You all are so kind and flexible. Zion, would that be okay by you? You get to choose our game next week and we can draw numbers to see who chooses the game the week after, I will keep track for us."

ZION: "Yeah!"

GROUP LEADER: "Great. Zion, I really like how you used your words AND practiced calming yourself down. That was so cool! We could figure out a solution because you spoke up for yourself AND listened to the group! We can figure so much out when we use our calm skills and talk to each other. Are you all ready to play Statue City?!"

You can see Zion's transferential response to the group. Zion, who feels forgotten at home in the wake of his mother's death, also feels left out during group processes. Zion is even able to identify being lost in the shuffle following his mother's death which shows useful insight crucial to the change process. **Highlighting the distinction between the client and therapist's individual experiences provides a window into client transference**, as is the case with Zion.

The clinician in the example above **recognized the transference reaction while encouraging both the leader-member dyad and the group as a whole to differentiate the experience through new lived and corrective experiences in the group here-and-now**. The clinician emphasized Zion's emotional reaction to the group and encouraged him to use an adaptive communication strategy (assertiveness/speaking up for himself) to self-regulate. Then, the group as a whole worked together to identify and agree on a solution.

Situations like the example above are commonplace in child groups. Managing transference also hinges on the successful resolution of the interactions. Clients must understand and work through their own individual transference responses elicited by the group and/or leaders. Groups are easy places to explore transference reactions, especially with group leaders. Children often place the issues they have with parents, caregivers, extended family or teachers onto clinicians who are able to see how they think and behave in everyday situations. **Ultimately, by working through transference reactions and resolving intrapersonal and interpersonal conflict through adaptive coping skills during group, skills can generalize into naturalistic settings**.

Exercise

Put yourself in this clinician's shoes for a moment. From the vignette, do you notice Zion's transference onto the group and group leader? How would you respond to Zion's initial reaction to the group choosing "Statue City"? Think for a moment about the child groups you run or would like to run. How does, or might, transference show up in those groups?

Clinician Countertransference

Countertransference is a very important and complex phenomenon in working with children. Historically, many clinicians understood their countertransference reactions as a way of understanding the ways that the patient needs us to be, a reflection of the internalized experiences with important others in the patient's life. This idea still holds true today. For example, a quiet group member may require the group leader to unconsciously direct a conversation with them.

Countertransference, like transference, is a window into the lives of our clients in-so-far as the social microcosm allows them to bring their authentic selves into group sessions. **The way we perceive clients, while filtered through our own lenses, provides information about our own lives and reactions. When combined with transference reactions from clients, we can identify how important others in a child's life might also feel**. Feeling frustrated with a child for not paying attention during a group conversation is likely a window into their parents' and teacher's experience. Group leaders can use these experiences and interpretations to positively impact group outcomes by using countertransference to inform clinical formulations, goals, objectives and interventions specific for each client.

Azima writing in Riester and Kraft (1986) defines countertransference as "The therapist's subjective, emotional and conflictual response to an individual patient or to the pressures of the group as a whole…which stretches horizontally in the present and vertically in time and integrates both intrapsychic and interpersonal phenomena" (pp. 141, 142). Azima's insights illuminate an integral concept for countertransference: Awareness of and management of countertransference is essential, both as a window into understanding the inner world of the client, but also as a means to prevent merely colluding in, acting out or repeating some reciprocal relationship with the client rather than helping the client pause and identify what the internalized needs, emotions and conflicts are.

The child group therapist is encouraged to engage in self-exploration and self-improvement as a way of preparing to deal with these countertransference reactions as they arise, deriving from the therapist needing to identify whether their feelings about a client stem from their own inner experiences or are induced by the client themselves.

Brems (2008) identifies four types of countertransference specific to children:

- **Issue-Specific Countertransference**, or clinician responses to client-specific behaviors, feelings, or needs which might not reflect the actual experience of the child. This type of countertransference is often a blend of transference and countertransference unique to the child-clinician dyad. For example, imagine a child talking about growing up in a neglectful household during a group session. A clinician with similar lived experiences may also share their story and assume their emotions are the same as the child's. If the issues presented by the child are too similar or threatening to their therapist's, it can create an unproductive countertransference response.
- **Stimulus-Specific Countertransference**, or clinician responses to non-clinical aspects of a client during treatment. The clinician may respond to similar, non-client children in the same way. For example, a client might remind a clinician of a childhood friend with whom the clinician regretted losing contact due to unresolved conflict. As such, the clinician may then respond in a way which involves this unresolved conflict regardless of the child's treatment needs. This overidentification with the client obscures an accurate understanding of the client and their experiences.
- **Trait-Specific Countertransference**, or habit-driven clinician responses which are global and occur inside and outside of therapy. The clinician's personality traits are relevant to trait-specific countertransference, since clinicians might respond to a certain

behavior regardless of setting. For example, an overly flexible clinician who avoids conflict may do so in group, regardless of the appropriateness of the situation. Thus, because of a particular personality trait of the therapist, the specifics and actuality of the client are lost.

•   **Child-Specific Countertransference**, or clinician responses which mirror most adults in the child's life. This type of countertransference is similar to Kernberg's (1965) identification of *objective countertransference*, or how most adults would react towards a client. In contrast, *subjective countertransference* is a reaction unique to the therapist. Client-specific countertransference is easily identified by cross-referencing impressions with parents, co-leaders, or teachers in the child's life. For example, if adults in the child's environment are often frustrated with oppositional behaviors which appear in group, it is specific to the child and not unique to the clinician.

In modern research, clinician reaction to child clients is an uncommon theoretical concept. Rasic (2010) summarizes three main reasons countertransference is not often talked about in child therapy literature:

1   The lack of operational definition and concurrent lack of measurement in an increasingly evidence-based therapy domain;
2   General discomfort in an honest evaluation of countertransference towards children who are a vulnerable population and
3   The abandonment of analyzing children apart from familial and social contexts, which was originally a heavily psychoanalytic construct.

As children are a vulnerable population with coinciding countertransference reactions to children and parents, it is easy to see why the subject is often excluded from study. Cultural values dictate a protective, loving attitude towards children who exist within complex systems, resulting in increasingly complicated countertransference. Because of these specific points, literature about countertransference within child therapy is scarce. This is to the detriment of child therapists as a whole who may gather significant information about clients by honestly examining their countertransference. Tsarkova (2015) discussed general countertransference reactions to children during play therapy while echoing both the lack of exploration into the subject and themes from Brems' and Rasic's work. She stated three major themes through exploratory qualitative research including feelings of frustration, feelings of uncertainty and complex countertransference feelings. Clinicians may feel uncomfortable when honestly exploring their countertransference to child clients because of their vulnerable status or because of their own lived childhood experiences.

As pointed out by Brems, self-awareness and willingness to self-explore open up issues related to therapists' own childhood experiences. Child groups bring to light leader-specific issues related to the leader's childhood (the 'subjective' countertransference reactions), caregiving experience and child-rearing practices. Gifted clinicians easily slip into countertransferential reactions with children and parents based on their own lived experiences – and in doing so react in self-serving or biased ways which do not best serve their clients. **Unpacking, exploring and processing lived experiences opens up clarity with interventions and here-and-now processing**. Child groups are uniquely positioned to process here-and-now experiences because of children's natural projection of feelings and lived experiences onto play scenarios.

Exploring countertransference is especially helpful with a co-leader. If using a co-leader model, unpacking interpersonal dynamics within a group allows double-checking of reactions in order to compare and contrast. If several members and leaders have the same reaction to a specific client, it is likely the reaction is clinically relevant and informative ('objective' countertransference). On the opposite side, if a leader has a specific countertransference reaction to a client that is not shared by others in the group, it is more likely the reaction is related to a leader-specific issue. Even as an individual leader, writing or intentionally noting countertransference reactions can be an effective way to explore group dynamics. **No matter the specific scenario, monitoring, reflecting on and identifying countertransference is beneficial to child groups**. As you are exploring countertransference, ask yourself some of the following self-reflection questions:

- What is my feeling towards this client? When do I feel this feeling in relation to this specific client?
- Do other people report having similar feelings to this client as I do? If yes, who? If no, what is their experience?
- What is my feeling to the group as a whole?
- What was my experience as a child at the age of this specific group?
- Are my experiences related to my inner world or truly elicited by the client?

Use of Self in Group Leadership

Use of self in therapy is an often-debated topic: How does one use themselves to develop authentic relationships within a group? What does it mean to "use yourself" as a group leader? What are the boundaries of self-disclosure and being "myself" while leading groups? Might genuine reactions or self-disclosures harm clients or the therapeutic work? What messages do you send as a group leader from the norms and rules you help create and enforce?

The most obvious (and infamous) answer is familiar to any clinician: *It depends*. **The use of self in group leadership requires a high level of clinical judgment and attunement to individual members and the group as a whole**. For example, a group leader may express basic emotional reactions to group behaviors as a way to provide feedback or encourage client emotional expression. However, this same behavior – leaders sharing emotional reactions to client behaviors – hinges completely on context. You might imagine scenarios where this is entirely appropriate and benefits the group, such as providing children interactive feedback on their behavior during the group. On the other hand, you can see how leader emotional disclosure may harm group processes, such as a group leader sharing strong emotional reactions during a support-only group. In this way, the use of self goes hand-in-hand with clinical judgment.

Another way of looking at the use of self in group leadership is therapist transparency and self-disclosure. Shechtman (2007) identified in her seminal work how self-disclosure can be particularly helpful with children. Child clients differ from adult clients with a forthright delivery of themselves and their experiences, often with only minimal tact. Children are honest, genuine and direct in their displays of feelings and thoughts. In short, you know where you stand with child clients. Children often expect such frank self-disclosure from others in their lives, including group leaders! One of the joys of working with children is being authentically ourselves, blending our professional knowledge and selves with honest expression of our personalities.

Self-disclosure, though not appropriate for every clinician in every setting, is a way to encourage and enrich the therapeutic relationship with children. After all, children do not attempt to hide themselves or their reactions to situations and stimuli in groups – often an assumption they make about others. Sharing your thoughts, reactions or experiences to members or the group as a whole has the added impact of developing the therapeutic relationship, especially with children. **Self-disclosure and transparency, when guided by therapeutic intent and focused on the growth of the client, can be normalizing and powerful**.

The historical roots of psychology are based in medical neutrality where clients would transfer themselves and their current working problems onto the therapist. Traditional psychoanalytic thought identifies resolution of transference as the most important healing factor. As psychotherapy has expanded and evolved, assuming an overly neutral stance ignores the stark reality that clinicians bring themselves into therapeutic work *every session*. The idea of true neutrality is a myth; as relational beings, we reveal who we are in many ways, consciously and unconsciously.

Office décor, dress, colloquialisms, waiting room magazines and even group rules reflect unique aspects or values of the clinician(s). The actual space clients enter is a physical representation of the clinician's use of self – and it sends clear messages to clients. Inclusive office décor sends signals of safety for clients from diverse backgrounds. An "All Gender" restroom sign reminds clients that their gender is respected. Diverse magazines, posters or books in the waiting room show clients that their identities are visible and valued. The same is true for the physical space of the group room. Carry this forward into group, one universal group rule is that insults or aggression towards an aspect of a member's identity will not be tolerated. This rule ultimately reflects an acceptance of diversity and an unwillingness to tolerate hateful speech or actions. In child and adolescent groups, this leads to a safe, brave exploratory group space in which to grow. All of these small rules and physical space setups are simple but clear representations of one's use of self that are not always considered. As with many aspects of group psychotherapy, intentionality is key!

Exercise

Every clinician reading this chapter is entirely different from the next. Consider these questions as ways to develop your own use of self:

- How am I as a person represented in my office environment?
- What do the group rules I create or co-create with my groups say about me?
- How am I represented in the way I talk to my clients? Do I feel true to myself when intervening with the majority of my clients? Why or why not?
- What is my use of self-disclosure with clients? Should I consider using more of my authentic reactions to clients during the group? Why or why not, and if yes, how?

Summary

In broad strokes, child groups uniquely pull playfulness, humor, flexibility, creativity, candidness and validation from the clinician. Intentionality is an important word in child group psychotherapy as it speaks to the challenge of balancing the authentic and the clinically deliberate. It is no small feat to be both authentic and clinical at the same time! Being intentional is sophisticated, advanced work which ultimately derives from self-exploration. However, the child group therapist benefits from the exploration of using one's self to augment theory and practice. In many ways, this is the art of psychotherapy: The blending of one's self into clinical theory in service of clients.

References

Altman, N., Briggs, R., Frankel, J., Gensler, D., & Pantone, P. (2002). *Relational child psychotherapy*. New York: Other Press.

Altman, N., Briggs, R., Frankel, J., Gensler, D., & Pantone, P. (2002). Transference and countertransference in child treatment. In N. Altman, R. Briggs, J. Frankel, D. Gensler, & P. Pantone (Eds.), *Relational child psychotherapy* (pp. 215–230). New York: Other Press.

Azima, F. J. (1986) Countertransference: In and beyond child group psychotherapy. In A. E. Riester, & I. A. Kraft (Eds.), *Child group psychotherapy: Future tense*. Madison, CT: International Universities Press, Inc.

Brems, C. (2008). *A comprehensive guide to child psychotherapy and counseling* (3rd ed.). Long Grove, IL: Waveland Press.

Bromfield, R. (2007). *Doing Child and adolescent therapy* (2nd ed.). Hoboken, NJ: Wiley.

Chiu, A. W., McLeod, B. D., Har, K., & Wood, J. J. (2009). Child–therapist alliance and clinical outcomes in cognitive behavioral therapy for child anxiety disorders. *Journal of Child Psychology & Psychiatry, 50*(6), 751–758. https://doi.org/10.1111/j.1469-7610.2008.01996.x

Corey, M. S., Corey, G., & Corey, C. (2018). *Groups: Process and practice*. Boston, MA: Cengage Learning.

Kernberg, O. (1965). Countertransference. *Journal of the American Psychoanalytical Association 13*, 38–56.

Lini, C., & Bertrando, P. (2020). Finding one's place: emotions and positioning in systemic- dialogical therapy. *Journal of Family Therapy, 42*(2), 204–221. https://doi.org/10.1111/1467-6427.12267

Rasic, D. (2010). Countertransference in child and adolescent psychiatry-a forgotten concept?. *Journal of the Canadian Academy of Child and Adolescent Psychiatry = Journal de l'Academie canadienne de psychiatrie de l'enfant et de l'adolescent, 19*(4), 249–254.

Rutan, J. S., Greene, L. R., & Kaklauskas, F. J. (2019). Basic leadership tasks. In F. J. Kaklauskas, & L. R. Greene (Eds.), *Core principles of group psychotherapy: An integrated theory, research, and practice training manual* (1st ed.) (pp. 111–121). New York: Routledge. https://doi.org/10.4324/9780429260803

Shechtman, Z. (2007). *Group Counseling and psychotherapy with children and adolescents theory, research, and practice: Theory, research, and practice* (1st ed.). New York: Routledge. https://doi.org/10.4324/9781315093369

Shechtman, Z., & Toren, Z. (2009). The effect of leader behavior on processes and outcomes in group counseling. *Group Dynamics: Theory, Research, and Practice, 13*(3), 218–233. https://doi.org/10.1037/a0015718

Smead, R. (1995). *Skills and techniques for group work with children and adolescents*. Champaign, IL: Research Press.

Tsarkova, A. (2015). *Exploring clinicians' experience of countertransference in play therapy*. Master's Thesis, Smith College, Northampton, MA. https://scholarworks.smith.edu/theses/669

Wanlass, J., Moreno, J. K., & Thomson, H. M. (2006). Group therapy for abused and neglected youth: therapeutic and child advocacy challenges. *Journal for Specialists in Group Work, 31*(4), 311–326.

Yalom, I. D., & Leszcz, M. (2020). *The theory and practice of group psychotherapy* (6th ed.). New York: Basic Books.

Yalom, I. D., & Leszcz, M. (2020). *The theory and practice of group psychotherapy* (6th ed.). New York: Basic Books. (Chapter 7: The therapist: transference and transparency).

6 Group Formation and Development

Tony L. Sheppard

Introduction

The best-executed groups are those in which therapists use theoretical grounding to answer practical questions about how to construct the group. Well-informed decisions regarding such factors as the physical layout of the room, the number of members to admit and what diagnoses to exclude can help to ensure the success of a therapy group. The group therapist must decide how best to structure the group sessions, how to balance the use of activities and group process and what topics or issues to include. While there are some accepted norms in terms of practical decisions, many depend upon the context of a given group. Even in situations where decisions are forced by the setting (e.g., a school that requires sessions to run for 30 minutes), the therapist's decisions on other factors can determine the degree of success of the group. Further, there are considerations related to involvement of parents and other collaterals in the group experience. Child group therapists must utilize their knowledge of child development and group therapy principles to ensure that growth and learning are maximized.

Children's therapy groups develop and change over time and thus it is important for the child group therapist to possess knowledge of the stages of group development. While there are similarities in stages of group development across child, adolescent and adult groups, the manner of presentation of developmental phenomena can be quite different. This chapter will review common practices, relevant research and theoretical principles that guide these important decisions. These considerations will assist the child group therapist in building successful groups.

Planning the Group

Decisions made prior to the start of the group can be critical to its success. Effective planning for the group can save the child group therapist a great deal of time in the long run. It can also ensure that the group develops in an effective manner, making it a better experience for its members.

Above all, planning entails a clear and explicit consideration of the goals of the group. A conceptualization of the therapeutic change processes will facilitate the achieving of those goals and considerations of group composition. Targeting the goals of the group to fit the particular needs of the individual members is of critical importance. Forming groups can be difficult, so it is important to plan for the process. From recruiting appropriate members, to the interventions used, to how the group will end, it is important that the therapists have a plan.

DOI: 10.4324/9781003189701-6

Group Proposal

Both Smead (1995) and Corey et al. (2018) recommend the use of a group proposal as a way of assisting the therapist in outlining the specifics of the group. In introducing the idea of a group proposal, Corey, Corey & Corey emphasize the fact that many excellent ideas for groups never come together due to a lack of preparation (p. 153). In addition to creating a streamlined purpose for the group, a group proposal is highly beneficial when marketing a group to other professionals so they know exactly what clients will make suitable group members. Smead (1995) recommends the following components in a proposal for a children's therapy group.

- **Description and rationale**
  - What is the purpose of the group?
  - Whose needs does it meet?
  - What topics will be explored?
- **Objectives**
  - Are treatment objectives clear?
  - Are they measurable so that the effectiveness of the group can be assessed?
  - Appropriate for the age and ability and developmental levels of the participants?
- **Logistics**
  - Who will lead the group?
  - How will group members be screened and selected?
  - When and where will the group meet?
  - How many will be admitted to the group?
- **Procedures**
  - What kind of techniques will be used?
  - How will confidentiality be explained and protected?
- **Evaluation**
  - How will the group leader determine whether a member has changed due to the group experience?
  - How will the group leader determine whether group objectives have been met?
  - What follow-up procedures will be used? (Summarized from Smead, 1995, pp. 25–27).

Group Composition Issues and Selecting Members

Group composition is an important consideration. **A primary question that the group therapist must ask focuses on homogeneity or heterogeneity of presenting problems**. Shechtman (2007) notes that experts tend to favor homogeneity for presenting problems in children's groups as exemplified in groups dealing with anger, divorce, ADHD, etc. She suggests that treating some sensitive issues such as coping with divorce, learning disorders, trauma or a specific identity background (such as LGBTQIA+ youth) might benefit from the sense of universality that emerges in a homogeneous group. Nevertheless, an argument can be made that heterogeneous groups for presenting issues will more readily facilitate the development of the social microcosm and more accurately reflect the environments in which children function (social groups, classrooms, sports teams, etc.), thus providing more opportunities to explore differences and diversity. The child group therapist will need to weigh these pros and cons and determine which kind of composition to construct. It should be noted that the literature on composition and selection doesn't reach consensus and that ultimately decisions are best made based upon clinical judgment.

Selecting members for the group is of critical importance to build groups that function well. It is important to determine inclusion and exclusion criteria for a given group. Tollison et al. (2007) recommend the following guidelines when considering children for membership in their groups (pp. 50, 51):

- The child's crisis level
  - Children who are actively in crisis benefit more from individual therapy
- Vulnerability of the child to disclosures that could be detrimental (e.g. discussion of suicide or self-harm)
- Willingness to work in a group setting
- Ability to take turns
- Ability to relate to others positively
- Level and type of differences in abilities

While this list is helpful on one level, it is important to keep in mind that some of these skills and abilities represent the actual work of the group. Therefore, these should be considered to exist on a continuum and that development of some of these capacities will be a focus of the group itself. Finally, Grunblatt (in Haen & Aronson, 2017) noted both social hunger or the desire for recognition and approval by others, and reciprocity or the mutual stimulation of ideas and feelings in a group setting as important to consider with regard to group composition.

When making decisions about how a given member will fit in a group, it is helpful to consider three realms of functioning: Cognitive, Interpersonal and Intrapersonal. These are defined as follows:

Cognitive-The overall cognitive functioning of the child. Includes measured IQ, cognitive flexibility and ability to comprehend the interactions of the group.

Interpersonal-The ability of the child to engage in relationships with others in the group. The degree to which they require assistance from others in order to accomplish this.

Intrapersonal-The awareness of the child of their own emotional responses to others. Their ability to manage emotional responses.

A continuum of functioning in each of these realms can be imagined (Figure 6.1).

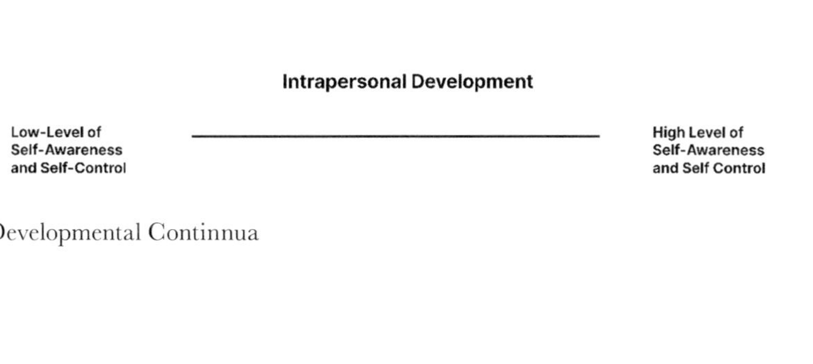

Cognitive Development

Concrete Thought ————————————— Abstract Thought

Interpersonal Development

Dependent upon others for connection ————————————— Connects with others independently

Intrapersonal Development

Low-Level of Self-Awareness and Self-Control ————————————— High Level of Self-Awareness and Self Control

Figure 6.1 Developmental Continnua

Consideration must be given to levels of functioning in these domains. Those children who lie far outside the average level of functioning for a given group would either need to be excluded from that group or a plan would need to be developed to accommodate their needs. While some differences in levels of functioning can be tolerated by a group, some cannot. For example, a group member who is almost totally reliant upon the group therapist in order to engage with others will likely not do well in a group in which most connect independently. Likewise, a child with very little impulse control will likely not fit well in a group of children who possess very good control over impulses. Ultimately, these decisions come down to the clinical judgment of the group therapist.

As will be discussed in the next section, pre-group interviews are a common way of gathering information regarding a group member's appropriateness for a given group. Shechtman (2007) cautions against excluding too many children based on an individual interview, as these may offer little indication of how successful the child will be in group therapy. She suggests that the primary value of the individual interview with the child is the promotion of therapist-child bonding. There is evidence that a meeting between the group leader and a potential group member can significantly improve the candidate's likelihood of follow-through and success in the group (Corey et al., 2018) and reduce a patient's resistance to group therapy (Crosby & Sabin, 1996).

Hurster in Haen & Aronson (2017) notes the ethical issues involved in group composition. He notes, "Inclusion and exclusion can be a complicated ethical dilemma in groups for youth because the emotional and cognitive maturity of some young group members can lead to overt expressions of intolerance and cruelty toward diverse members" (p. 69). On the other hand, the group therapist grapples with issues of denying needed care to potential members of the group. This leads the therapist to consider the balance of what is greater for the group vs. the individual. In general, if a child is accepted into a group who is divergent from others in that group in the realms of intrapersonal, cognitive or interpersonal functioning, the group leader must be certain that they can scaffold that child enough so that their involvement in the group is successful.

Many therapists likely err on the side of inclusion in these situations. When this occurs, there is a need to support that group member so that they can function in the group to the best of their current ability. The following case example is meant to illustrate some of the ways this might occur in a group setting.

Jeff is a 9-year-old male who is being considered for involvement in a heterogeneous co-ed group for children ages 9–11. Jeff has a diagnosis of Attention Deficit Hyperactivity Disorder, Combined Type for which he is currently not medicated. He is home-schooled and has very little interaction with other children other than his younger sister, who has a diagnosis of Autism Spectrum Disorder. Jeff functions generally at or above the overall level of the group cognitively.

However, with regard to his emotional and self-awareness (intrapersonal functioning) and his interpersonal functioning, he is significantly below the general level of the group. The group co-leaders are of the opinion that while Jeff's presentation diverges from that of the overall group, they can sufficiently support and scaffold Jeff such that he can participate successfully in the group.

The co-leaders agree to put the following into place to ensure Jeff's success in the group:

- Talk with Jeff's mother about considering medication to address his significant symptoms of ADHD.
- Create group goals related to Jeff's ADHD while also affirming his neurodivergence in a supportive manner.
- Provide Jeff with fidget toys with which he can play during group sessions to assist him with some of his excess energy.

- Utilize confrontation in a supportive manner to address behaviors that are problematic in the group.
  - Redirect Jeff when he is out of his seat, not keeping his hands and feet to himself, etc.
  - Redirect Jeff when he engages in off-topic verbalizations
  - Redirect Jeff when he engages in silly behavior that is off task
- Pair Jeff with a 'group buddy' who is an established member of the group to help him focus and remain on task.
- Conduct a group session on I-Statements so that all group members are empowered with a way to confront each other in a supportive and healthy manner.
- Model the use of I-Statements in interactions with Jeff
  - E.g., "Jeff, I get annoyed when you respond to our problem solving activity with silly solutions. I'd like for you to give us some serious solutions to the problem. If you don't have any, maybe you could ask others for help."

Pre-group Preparation

There is general agreement that a pre-group meeting and orientation is beneficial prior to introducing a child into a therapy group. Grunblatt in Haen & Aronson (2017) notes that this meeting "is intended to promote comfort and familiarity for both parent and young person" (p. 22). This author goes on to suggest that this screening also affords the therapist the opportunity to observe the child in interaction with caregivers. Finally, it is noted to offer an opportunity to orient the child to the group therapy process. Smead (1995) recommends an individual interview that allows for "privacy and disclosure on the child's part as well as for you (therapist) to focus in on that child to get a reading on his or her suitability for the group" (p. 38).

Corey et al. (2018) note the importance of pre-group preparation stating,

> The overwhelming consensus is that preparation positively affects both early therapeutic processes and later client involvement…Pre group preparation is positively associated with group cohesion and members' satisfaction with their experience; preparing members for a group experience is a key aspect of informed consent
>
> (p. 163).

It is essential that the group therapist conduct a pre-group interview of some type with children before they enter a group.

Brabender (2002) notes the following means of obtaining information about a prospective group member in determining their appropriateness for the group:

- Interviewing
- Direct Observation of Group Behavior (e.g., classroom or small group observation)
- Personality Assessment Tools

Obviously, some of these tasks will involve the group member and others will involve the parents, guardians, or caregivers of the child.

With regard to group preparation, Rutan et al. (2014) note the following important points:

- Building a positive emotional bond and positive working alliance with the patient in the screening session and especially the early stages of the group
- Informing the patient about the nature of the group
- Reviewing the group agreements

- Reviewing logistical information (e.g., time and location of the group)
- Exploring and addressing assumptions, anxieties and resistances

While these points come from an adult focused perspective on groups, the spirit behind them applies very well to children and their guardians. After all, child group clinicians are working with caregivers and clients and need a strong relational foundation with both. Obviously, with children, information about the group is to be presented in a developmentally appropriate manner that they can understand and integrate into their experiences.

Pre-group meetings are often the best time to review policies in the group with guardians. Issues that might be addressed at this time include:

- Payment
- Time and length of group sessions
- Expectations for change
- The importance of working toward goals at home
- The importance of consistent attendance in the group
- Missed appointments/cancellations
- Termination/withdrawal from group

A sample structure for a pre-group meeting is presented below:
Meet with caregivers

- Review confidentiality, obtain consent forms and review payment information
- Get their input on the presenting problem
- Review the main focus areas of the group
- Review the procedures for parent involvement in the group
- Confirm when child will begin group sessions

Meet with caregivers and the child

- Review confidentiality
- Prompt for any questions about group sessions
- Observe how parents and child interact with each other

Meet with the child

- Get their input on the presenting problem and get to know them- what they like/dislike, how they feel about group
- Review the main focus areas of the group
- Tell them what to expect in their first group session
    o Introductions
    o Talk as much as you feel comfortable talking
- Answer their questions and address concerns or anxieties, overtly expressed or implied
- Ask about the child's identities and affirm that the group is welcoming to those with differing identities
- Show them the group room
- General rapport-building/getting to know the child's hobbies and interests
- Let them know you're glad they're joining the group!

An example of the selection and screening procedures for our practice follows. The practice offers multiple groups for children on an ongoing basis:

Screening: Office staff use a standardized questionnaire to obtain information on the presenting issues for the child. This information is then presented to the group staff in a weekly staffing meeting. Group leaders discuss the appropriateness of this member for the groups that are offered. If slots are available for an appropriate group, then that person is scheduled for a group intake with one of the group leaders. Decisions regarding placement in a group are made collaboratively between the group leader and the guardian/s.

Assessment: Caregivers of the child are asked to complete a multi-informant rating scale that screens for a number of behavioral health diagnoses for the child. This assists the group leaders in knowing the specific challenges faced by the child and their family.

Interview: The interview proceeds as follows:

15–20 Minutes   Meet with caregivers

- Very briefly review the results of the Multi-Informant Rating Scale or other assessment
- Solicit their input on the presenting problem
- Review the Three Main Focus Areas of Group
  - Self-Regulation-Knowing your own emotions and learning to manage them
  - Interpersonal/Social Skills-Dealing with others effectively
  - Self-Esteem-Building a sense of self-confidence
- Review the Parent Feedback Schedule
  - We reach out every 15 weeks to check in on progress
  - This is how we determine how long an individual spends in group
  - They are welcome to contact the group leaders at any time with questions or concerns
- Provide parents/guardians with printed information about the group including the following:
  - Group Orientation Guide with an overview of broad goals of the group
  - Fee Schedule/Group Meeting Schedule
  - Information Sheets on
    - Goal Setting that reviews the types of goals that are appropriate for the group and how goals are generally identified
    - Outside Contact Rules outlining guidelines for when and how it is appropriate for group members to have contact outside the group
- Complete and send any Releases of Information that are needed (e.g. teachers, pediatrician, psychiatrist, therapist, etc.)
- Confirm when the child will begin group sessions

10 Minutes   Meet with parent/s or guardian and the child

- Review confidentiality
- Prompt for any questions about group sessions
- Ask questions about mood/sleep/appetite
- Observe how parents and child interact with each other

20 Minutes   Meet with the child

- Ensure that they know what is being discussed
  - Some parents don't tell their children much about the appointment

- Get their input on the presenting problem and get to know them – what they like/dislike, how they feel about group including their worries and resistances to joining the group
- Review the Three Main Focus Areas of Group
  - Knowing your own feelings and learning to manage them
  - Learning how to deal with others and differences effectively
  - Building a sense of self-confidence/Believing in yourself
- Tell them what to expect in their first group session
  - Introductions
  - Learning time
  - Game time
  - Talk as much as you feel comfortable talking
- Help the child to identify some goals for the group. Often, it is helpful to frame this as "what would you like to learn in the group?" or "what would you like to get better at in the group?"
  - See the Group Goals Menu in Chapter 8 of this book
- Let them know you're glad they're joining the group!

Time Formats

There are a number of decisions that need to be made when planning a group with regard to time. The first relates to the length of the group sessions themselves. Most outpatient therapy groups use 60- or 90-minute formats. Some specialized formats have sessions of variable durations. Inpatient groups may be shorter due to the decreased attention capacity of children in acute distress. School-based groups may use shorter formats so as not to impinge upon instruction time. Youth programs (summer camps, day therapy programs, etc.) may meet for longer periods of time. However, these group-based programs often schedule activities in 30–90-minute blocks of time. **Decisions about the duration of group sessions should be made based upon the needs and capacities of the children**. The following factors must be considered:

- **Age**: Younger children often have shorter attention spans
- **Clinical issues**: Children will have varying degrees of frustration tolerance and attention span based upon their diagnoses and presenting problems
- **Structure of the group sessions**: Need to assess sufficient time for structured work and process exploration. Sessions that have less structured time built in (play time, games, etc.) can often run longer than those that are very structured

Whatever the time duration of group sessions, it is important to adhere to that. Starting and ending on time helps to establish trust and cohesion in the group. Children and caregivers are dependent on the predictability of group sessions adhering to specific timelines, especially given how spending too much time can infringe upon other activities regardless of setting.

Another important decision that the group therapist must consider with regard to timing of the group has to do with time-limited groups versus open-ended groups. **Time-limited groups meet for a specified number of sessions and typically are closed to new members once the group begins since there is usually a preplanned sequence of topics to be addressed**. Advantages to this format include fewer dropouts since the duration of the group is determined and shorter than an open-ended group. Additionally, these groups tend to be planned from the beginning so that the work may be more focused. In other words, topics and activities are planned and likely adhered to lending more focus to the sessions. This might serve to enhance group cohesion since there is a sense that "we're all in this together for the duration of the group." Disadvantages to a time-limited group model include a potential lack of time for a true process focus. Secondly, due to time limits, these groups may not progress through all the group stages.

Open-ended Groups (also referred to as continuous groups) meet on an ongoing basis and typically accept new members as older members drop out or complete the group. This format has the advantage that the group will tend to progress through the different stages of group development. Also, children can learn how to welcome new members to the group as well as how to say goodbye to those who leave the group. Further, there is benefit in meeting and being accepted by new people as they enter the group. This time format often does permit a focus on group process in that there may be less pressure on the group leader/s to cover topical material. Potential disadvantages to open-ended groups are that they can lose focus over the course of time. Also, dropout rates can be higher since there is often no set end point for treatment.

Structure of the Sessions

The structure of group sessions is a very important consideration for the therapist as they imagine their group. A continuum of structure to child groups can be imagined. At the less structured end of this continuum is Slavson's activity group therapy. In this model, it was believed that children needed a "permissive environment" to work out their frustration and drives. During early stages of groups, a permissive stance is taken with "diffuse hilarity and wild behavior" (Slavson, in Riester & Kraft, 1986, pp. 20, 21). This stance is taken to allow children to let off steam. On the other end of this continuum, the model discussed by Corey et al. (2015) urges group leaders to provide much more structured in their approach, particularly at the beginning of a group, by establishing and reinforcing norms and maintaining focus on therapeutic work. Group leaders are called upon to determine the degree of structure in their groups using clinical judgment.

There are pitfalls to both over and under-structuring group sessions. Group sessions that are overly structured tend to limit opportunities to explore the social microcosm of the group. Under-structured sessions can become overly chaotic and not adequately address group goals.

Sample group sessions for an hour-long child therapy group:

Check-in and warm-up activity (10 minutes)
Review of group goals (10 minutes)
Structured therapeutic activity (20 minutes)
Goal progress review and Goal setting for the next session based upon activity (10 minutes)
Review of the session/rewards (10 minutes)

Children can only handle so much content in a given session. While this sample may go exactly as planned, group therapists must flexibly adapt to the group's needs. If over time the group is unsuccessful with too much structure, it may be helpful to reduce the amount of structured activities or vice versa for groups with too little structure.

Physical Configuration of the Setting

The physical configuration of the setting is an important consideration in group therapy. This is highly dependent upon the objectives, composition and type of group. General requirements for the group space include the following:

- The room or space provides adequate privacy for conducting the sessions.
  - Free from interruptions or distractions from outside the room
  - Away from caregivers to maintain privacy
- It is welcoming to children in its décor, tone and atmosphere.
  - Furnishings are appropriate for children. Highly valuable furnishings and decor would best be left out of this space to ensure they are not damaged or broken during group activities.
- The space is physically safe for children, free from items that could be harmful.
  - No unsafe cleaning materials, sharp items, dangerous kitchen utensils, etc.
- Perhaps most important, a space that provides a sense of safety, containment and security.

The degree of structure to the sessions will impact the physical arrangements. Some examples of this are:

Seating

More structured: Tables and chairs with assigned seating
Less structured: Pillows, sofas, and beanbag chairs

Toys

More structured: Room contains no toys, or toys are in a designated space with rules governing their use.
Less structured: Toys are in the group area with few rules governing their use.

Snacks

More structured: Snacks are served by group leaders or by the children according to group norms and rules, or no snacks at all.
Less structured: Snacks are available to children when they enter the group space.

Building Diverse and Culturally Consonant Groups

Diversity in group composition often deals with decisions around gender, ethnicity and other cultural considerations. When the social microcosm proposed by Yalom and Leszcz (2020) is considered, heterogeneity in group composition is preferred. In a general sense, **groups with diversity with regard to gender and other factors will better resemble the social settings within which children function**. That said, the child group therapist must take into account several factors in making decisions about the composition and functioning of their groups.

Child group therapists must take into account the impact of the broader culture (generally speaking of Western Judeo-Christian society) on subcultures from which children present. Kamsani et al. in Haen & Aronson (2017) note that groups will develop their own cultures that are likely influenced by the cultures from which their members come. **Child therapists must be mindful of client culture and incorporate it into group activities in order to foster client identity development**.

Further, Steen, Vanatta & Liu (in Haen & Aronson, 2017) note that the culturally adaptive therapist must consider how cultures impact the child's ability to engage in the group and even their presenting issues and how they are conceptualized.

Situations that would require specific cultural adaptations could include the following:

- A child from a rural area joining a group of children from an urban setting
- A Muslim-identified child joining a group of predominantly Jewish-identified children
- A Black-identified child joining a group of mostly White-identified children
- An Atheist-identified child joining a group of mostly Christian identified children
- A Gay-identified child joining a group of predominantly straight-identified children

Discussing identity differences and the impact on clients before joining a group allows for open exploration of culture. Identity salience is important to making decisions about goodness of fit for group. For example, if a faith-based group is located within a synagogue and comprised entirely of Jewish members, a Christian member would not likely be a good fit. While this point may seem obvious, **it is important for group leaders to actively attend to client culture and how it fits with the individual cultural origins of other members**.

A useful construct to consider when making decisions regarding group composition is *Frustration Tolerance*. Frustration Tolerance is defined as the capacity of the child for coping with the frustration inherent in group process. This frustration may result from:

- Being redirected by the group leader/s.
- Having one's views challenged.
- Waiting one's turn in an activity.
- Listening to others.
- Sharing the resources of the group.
- Being asked to delay gratification.
- Feeling different from the others in the group.

In order to be successful in a therapy group, children need a moderate degree of frustration tolerance. Children who do not possess at least a moderate degree of frustration tolerance should work on developing it in individual therapy prior to joining a group.

Dealing with Dropouts

Child group therapists are advised to consider actions that will prevent dropouts from their groups. Good screening procedures, clarity regarding goals and alliance building and ensuring that cohesion develops in groups all work to prevent premature dropouts from the group. Further, regular meetings with parents and/or guardians help to ensure alignment of goals and to make regular decisions regarding treatment.

- Inevitably even with the aforementioned factors in place, children will drop out of groups. Smead (1995) recommends, when possible, having a child attend a final session in order to say goodbye and to inform the group of their departure. There may be a need to process dropouts with the remaining children. Remaining members may need some closure on this. If attending a final session is not possible, processing the impacts of the lost member on the group and its members is important. Additionally, writing a goodbye letter to the departed member could help bring some closure and decrease the sense of broken container.

Stages of Group

There are a number of terms used to describe the stages of development in a therapy group. Tuckman (1965) proposed the following stages:

- Forming
- Storming
- Norming
- Performing

Corey et al. (2015) propose the following stages:

- Initial stage
- Transition stage
- Working stage
- Final stage

Many group stage theories encapsulate the general process of group members getting to know each other, testing vulnerability, creating a cohesive working environment and terminating. The stages proposed by Corey et al. (2015) have become the most widely accepted and will be used in describing the characteristics of each stage, as applied to a time-limited group.

Initial Stage

During the initial stage of the group, the basic task is establishing trust (Corey et al., 2015, p. 72). Other tasks that these authors note are Identifying and dealing with fears (pp. 75, 76) and Addressing Resistance and Modeling (pp. 76, 77). Shechtman (2007) notes the following tasks for group leaders in the initial stages of a group:

- Forming relationships
  - Introductions
  - Creating a familiar environment
- Developing a language of feelings
  - Assisting children in learning to talk about their emotions
- Establishing constructive group norms
- Providing a sense of security

A number of authors stress the importance of setting clear and agreed upon goals during this stage of the group (Bernard et al., 20008; Corey et al., 2018; Yalom & Leszcz, 2020).

The following represents a sample of topics to be covered and activities that nurture a group's development during the initial stage.

Session One: Introductions of group members using creative means and games.
- Members share things about themselves such as their favorite activities and foods, where they go to school, pets that they have, information about their families, something funny they've watched recently, a talent they have, etc.
- Children are engaged in games and activities that allow them to get to know each other such as Whonu from Cranium, Apples to Apples, and Spectrogram and Sociogram exercises such as a step-in-circle.

Session Two: Using the Group Goals Menu (see Chapter 8 of this book) to help group members identify individual goals. Members can be engaged in discussion about group goals and norms. They could make posters or use a whiteboard to brainstorm group norms (e.g. no name calling, listen when others are talking, follow directions, etc.).

Session Three: Group members are encouraged to learn about emotions and how they feel in our bodies and how they look. Such an activity can actually be spread out over multiple sessions with a focus on different feelings each session. Games such as emotions charades can help to reinforce this work.

Session Four: Group members are encouraged to talk about their feelings about the group. This helps to gauge how members are responding to the group overall and to allow them to express residual fears and anxieties. Simply asking members to express one thing they like about the group and one thing they don't like can be powerful. This allows members to express themselves and it also sets a norm of openness and honesty in the group. Members could be engaged in a group activity that promotes group cohesion such as producing a group skit or music video or making a group poster or art project.

Transition Stage

Corey et al. (2018) note characteristics of the transition stage (pp. 173–183):

- Anxiety
  - Fear of sounding stupid
  - Fear of losing control
  - Fear of being misunderstood
  - Fear of being rejected
  - Fear of not knowing what is expected
- The testing process and building trust
  - When trust is low, members may be more tentative while testing the climate.
  - When trust is established, members will begin to take more risks.
- Defensiveness and resistance
  - Members may rely on skills that they typically use in stressful situations.
- Struggle for control
  - Characteristic behaviors may include:
    - Competition
    - Rivalry
    - Jockeying for position
    - Jealousness
- Conflict
  - There is a tendency to avoid conflict in groups, but this must be worked through for the group to be productive
- Challenges to the group leader

Corey et al. (2018) note the importance of the leader's reactions to resistance. These authors emphasize helping the client to better understand the reasons for their resistance rather than responding based upon our own (therapist's) feelings about this.

When considering the differences in the ways this stage manifests itself in adults versus children, Smead (1995) notes that children may struggle less with trust than adults, moving more quickly into the working stage. Shechtman (2007) summarizes the research to explain four primary types of resistance shown by children in this stage of a group (p. 92). These are listed in order from most to least prevalent:

- Refusal to respond
- Distracting behavior

- Outburst of anger
- Verbal aggression

The following vignette demonstrates some issues that might arise in a children's therapy group during the transition stage of the group.

Group leaders have noticed as the group has progressed into its fifth and sixth sessions that the members are becoming more challenging. Some group members are expressing frustration with others in the group for their off-task behavior. Group members argue a lot with each other. They are resisting the use of I-Statements, instead reverting back to blaming each other. Some members refuse to engage in games and activities calling them "dumb" and "boring." There is more off-task behavior in the group that takes the form of silliness (e.g. members making noises, passing gas in the room and being generally emotionally reactive to the others in the group and with the group leaders).

The group leaders respond with supportive confrontation and redirection of these behaviors. Sometimes interpretations are made that help members to gain better insight into the motivations behind their behavior. Group norms and rules are firmly but supportively upheld by the group leaders. These interventions are combined with some behavior modification strategies (e.g. stamps for positive and pro-social behaviors, removal of privileges for negative behaviors) to assist members in adjusting to this stage of the group.

Group leaders focus on helping members to understand the impacts of their behaviors and to the extent appropriate some of the motivations behind this. Activities, both cognitive and experiential, are employed to assist members in reinforcing the norms and rules of the group. Particular emphasis is placed on activities that permit members to regulate their emotions and learn to deal with frustrations in positive ways. Concurrent with this, emphasis is placed upon developing group cohesion. Activities are offered that help the group to come together in common goals rather than fragmenting.

Working Stage

Corey et al. (2018) describe the working stage as being "characterized by the commitment of members to explore significant problems they bring to the sessions and by their attention to the dynamics within the group" (p. 276). Depending on the length and open/closed nature of the group, there may be considerable time spent in this stage. Smead (1995) notes the following behaviors and situations in the working stage with children:

- Children coming to group saying that they are practicing the new skills and behaviors they learned in the group in other situations
- Children following the norms set in the group
- Children's ability to be more immediate and deal with the here-and-now context of things that happen in the group
- Children's ability to articulate their plans and goals
- Children's ability to ask for help from other group members and profit from feedback. (p. 64)

Shechtman (2007) notes that in this stage children are able to (p. 97):

- Share personal information
- Listen to one another
- Be supportive of others' attempts to progress
- Express positive and negative feelings

- Ask for help
- Help other participants process their issues by:
  ○ Questioning
  ○ Providing honest feedback
  ○ Contributing to their self-understanding and insight
- Be more immediate and deal with the here-and-now context of things that happen in the group

The following vignette offers insight into how a group might present during the working stage. Imagine members of the group are engaged in a Lego activity that focuses on creativity, self-confidence and sharing. One member, Sophia, is frustrated that other members are "taking all the good Legos." She breaks her Lego creation apart and tosses it into the bin full of Legos and says, "I quit. They're getting all the good pieces and I can't build my house." The group leader encourages Sophia to breathe and relax and take a minute to calm down. Others in the group suggest that she practice "Oh Well!," a letting go strategy that the group learned a few sessions ago. Sophia takes a deep breath and says, "Oh Well. I can let it go." The group is engaged in problem solving with her to assist her in overcoming her strong feelings about the Legos. She eventually comes back to the group with the help and support of the group leaders and other members and completes her "house." She is able to express that it's not perfect because she couldn't have all the pieces she wanted, but that this is "OK." Other members of the group congratulate her on practicing her skills in the group.

Final Stage

Corey et al. (2018) note that it is important, during this stage, to help members consolidate learning that has occurred in the group. Group leaders must consider how to encourage members to carry their learning further. These authors point out that termination of the group experience involves a grieving process as well. This process may trigger feelings related to other losses members have experienced. Since children often do not always possess the developmental capacity and self-awareness to verbally process all of the emotions triggered by termination of the group experience, they may be expressed behaviorally.

Shechtman (2007) notes the following overall objectives of the final or termination stage of a group:

- Dealing with Loss and Separation
- Parting through Positive Feedback
- Evaluating Growth In and Out of the Group
- Evaluating the Group Experience
- Making Plans for the Future
- Separation from the Group Leader

To the degree that children lack self-expression abilities and frustration tolerance, there should be additional structure to termination experiences. This structure helps children to express the emotion of saying goodbye and ensures that they have a positive experience with the termination of the group. Group leaders are cautioned to never trust indifference. All children have feelings about leaving a group of which they have been a part. Smead (1995) offers a number of closing rituals for children's groups including:

- Thank-you cards
- Group poem
- A party or celebration

Other ideas for ending rituals include:

- **A Letter to Myself** – Members are encouraged to list things they learned in the group in a letter format. The group leader then mails them their letter a few weeks after the group ends or that member terminates from the group.
- **Certificates** – Group members are given a certificate for completion of their participation in the group.
- **Posters** – Group members sign and/or draw pictures on a poster that is then given to the departing member or members.
- **Imaginary Present Game** – Group members present each other with imaginary presents (Shechtman, 2007).
- **Free time to Reminisce about the group** (Corey et al., 2018).
- **Goodbye Packets** – Using practice and outside resources to continue care post-group.

Employing Multiple Learning Modalities

When working with children it is important to engage multiple learning modalities for optimal growth, development and change in the group process. As discussed in the development chapter, children require various methods such as play to learn group messages. Gardner's Theory of Multiple Intelligences recognizes that people learn in very different ways. Group leaders should consider the different learning styles and needs of children when conducting groups. Interventions that allow for various ways of learning and experiencing should be integrated into all therapy groups.

The child group therapist is encouraged to consider these multiple intelligences when planning and executing group activities:

- Linguistic
- Logical/mathematical
- Musical
- Spatial
- Kinesthetic

Examples will be given in Chapter 8 of the current text for engaging the different intelligences in planning group activities.

Summary

Planning for groups is an important part of their success. A group proposal can guide child group therapists in thinking through important aspects of the group prior to its launch. As the child group therapist plans for their groups, an awareness of group development will serve them well. While groups develop in their own unique and nuanced ways, there are accepted stages that groups go through in their development. Consideration of the needs of the group and its members at these various stages is critical to the group's success!

Questions for Discussion and Review

1   What are the elements of a good *group proposal*? Discuss ways that a *group proposal* could be used in different settings (e.g., planning, securing funding, informing others).

2   Discuss important factors for selecting members for a group. Consider ways of assessing these in a screening session or intake.

3   Presentation of the characteristics of *group stages* with children is influenced by their developmental level and is often seen through behavior. Discuss ways that these characteristics differ in children's groups from that seen in adult groups.

4   This book recommends that issues around diversity become part of the subculture of the group meaning that these issues are frequently openly processed in groups. Consider the implications and limits of this approach:

   a   Are there issues that are not appropriate to process?

   b   Under what circumstances would processing not be appropriate?

   c   What safeguards should group therapists put in place regarding this?

   d   When is parental consent needed or when should parents be made aware that a sensitive issue has been processed?

   e   How might therapist worldview (e.g. values, beliefs and even counter transference) impact such processing?

5   Choose a population or presenting issue (e.g., children of divorce, ADHD, anxiety) and consider the following with regard to proposing a group focusing on it. Discuss the following in relation to the group:

   a   Length of the sessions

   b   Duration (open-ended versus time-limited)

   c   Structure of the sessions

   d   Physical configuration of the space

   e   Activities and interventions

   f   Working systemically

Critical Thinking Activity: Group Composition Exercise

In this exercise, learners will be asked to make decisions regarding inclusion or exclusion of members from a forming group. Beyond that, learners are asked to consider concerns as they form each group. Learners should consider each person's intersecting identities as they impact the person entering the group.

The group: A group for children with social skills deficits that will run throughout the school year.

*   Brent – A 9-year-old White boy diagnosed with Bipolar Disorder. Brent experiences tantrums at home and at school that can last for over an hour. Brent likes group activities and seems drawn to others in his class. He attends the same school as Connie.

*   William – An 8-year-old Japanese American boy who is bullied by others at school. He is very shy and slow to warm up. William is diagnosed with Generalized Anxiety Disorder and stated that his biggest worry is about being in the group is "someone getting mad and throwing things."

*   Connie – A 10-year-old Black girl who is one of the brightest students in her school. Connie also identifies as gay. She is described by her mother as "loud and not getting social cues." She is diagnosed with Autism Spectrum Disorder, Level 1. She attends the same school as Brent.

- Dotti – A highly anxious 9-year-old White Jewish girl. She is diagnosed with Social Anxiety Disorder. She sometimes obsesses "for days" over a simple interaction with a peer. She is home-schooled after a failed attempt at attending a small local Jewish day-school. Her anxiety became unmanageable. She is excited about joining a group of other kids.
- Susan – A 10-year-old White girl diagnosed with Autism Spectrum Disorder, Level 1. Susan has no friends and is teased relentlessly at school. She recently attended a group for children diagnosed with Autism, but refused to go back due to feeling she didn't identify with that group.
- Sean – An 8-year-old White boy who is being discharged from an inpatient facility. He has a diagnosis of Disruptive Mood Dysregulation Disorder. He was hospitalized after picking up a chair and threatening to throw it at peers in his classroom. His hospital social worker says he's "improved greatly" on medications. Sean did not do well in group therapy while he was in the hospital.
- Ernie – A Latinx boy who is 9 and presents with a good deal of hyperactivity. He is diagnosed with Attention Deficit Hyperactivity Disorder, Combined Type. Ernie has never been in therapy according to his parents. They didn't bring him to the initial appointment, stating that "he would get bored and leave." Ernie doesn't relate well to other kids at school. He tends to "ignore them."
- Marissa – A very quiet and shy 12-year-old Chinese-American girl who will only talk with her mouth covered. She has been in individual therapy for 3 months with another therapist with no significant gains. She is diagnosed with Social Anxiety Disorder. During the intake, she would not make eye contact with or talk to the therapist.
- Sal – A 7-year-old Black boy who has been diagnosed with Attention Deficit Hyperactivity Disorder, Combined Type and Oppositional Defiant Disorder. He has been referred for group therapy by his individual therapist to develop social skills. He tends to play best with the kids in pre-school and kindergarten at his school even though he's in first grade. Sal is excited about joining a group, but his parents are fearful that he will "learn bad behaviors from the other kids."

What preparation might be needed and what factors might the group therapist need to consider with regard to preparation for each member? What questions would the group therapist ask each participant in order to assess their readiness and appropriateness for the group? Are there parts of the person's presentation that could represent barriers in their relating to others in the group as the group leaders consider how to build cohesion? Finally, if children are not included in the group, the learner should designate a form of treatment that would be appropriate for that individual and consider how to best communicate that decision to prevent harm.

References

Aronson, S., & Haen, C. (2017). *Handbook of child and adolescent group therapy: A practitioner's reference*. New York: Routledge.

Bernard, H., Burlingame, G., Flores, P., Greene, L., Joyce, A., Kobos, J. C., Leszcz, M., MacNair-Semands, R. R., Piper, W. E., McEneaney, A. M., & Feirman, D. (2008). Clinical practice guidelines for group psychotherapy. *International Journal of Group Psychotherapy*, *58*(4), 455–542. https://doi.org/10.1521/ijgp.2008.58.4.455

Brabender, V. (2002). *Introduction to group therapy*. Hoboken, NJ: Wiley.

Corey, G., Corey, M. S., Callahan, P., & Russell, J. M. (2015). *Group techniques*. Boston, MA: Cengage Learning.

Corey, M. S., Corey, G., & Corey, C. (2018). *Groups: Process and practice*. Boston, MA: Cengage Learning.

Crosby, G., & Sabin, J. E. (1996). A planning checklist for establishing time-limited psychotherapy groups. *Psychiatric Services, 47*(1), 25–26. https://doi.org/10.1176/ps.47.1.25

Haen, C., & Aronson, S. (2017). *Handbook of child and adolescent group therapy: A practitioner's reference* (pp. 193–202). New York, NY: Routledge.

Riester, A. E., & Kraft, I. A. (1986). *Child group psychotherapy: Future tense*. Madison, CT: International Universities Press.

Rutan, J. S., Stone, W. N., & Shay, J. J. (2014). *Psychodynamic group psychotherapy* (5th ed.). New York: The Guilford Press.

Shechtman, Z. (2007). *Group counseling and psychotherapy with children and adolescents: Theory, research, and Practice*. New York: Routledge.

Smead, R. (1995). *Skills and techniques for group work with Children and adolescents*. Champaign, IL: Research Press.

Tollison, P. K., Synatschk, K. O., & Synatschk, C. (2007). *Sos!: A practical guide for leading solution-focused groups with Kids K-12*. Austin, TX: PRO-ED.

Tuckman, B. W. (1965). Developmental sequence in small groups. *Psychological Bulletin, 63*(6), 384–399. doi:10.1037/h0022100. PMID 14314073

Yalom, I. D., & Leszcz, M. (2020). *The theory and practice of group psychotherapy*. New York: Basic Books.

7 Ethical Concerns in Groups with Children

Zachary J. Thieneman

Introduction

Ethics is an integral part of clinical practice yet frequently takes a back seat to theory and practice. In reality, ethics combines practice and morality for the overall safety of the public. It is an overtly critical part of treatment based in a clinician's individual cultural morality. **Ethical practice is especially important working with children, who are a protected and vulnerable population**.

Children bring unique challenges to ethical practice. Apart from the ethics of working with people across the age span such as honoring diversity, confidentiality and beneficence, ethical components unique to child treatment include morality-based foundations of ethics principles, confidentiality with caregivers, behavior management strategies and accountability strategies. Beyond the typical ethical dilemmas faced by mental health clinicians, children add a layer of systemic and developmental complexity which child clinicians must be aware of. Each of these will be discussed in isolation and their relevance to child treatment to prepare clinicians for the ethical scenarios which will be encountered during everyday practice. Throughout this chapter, short examples will be used to illustrate ethical points. They are also useful in guiding clinicians through common ethical scenarios in child group practice. By thoughtfully considering them, therapists may also find them useful when planning or implementing a child group!

Starting Points for Ethical Practice

Every professional mental health organization offers guidelines on ethical behaviors and practice. Each provides basic starting points for ethical treatment. They offer guideposts to continually monitor and integrate into daily practice which serve as boundaries for interventions. Like much research and information in the broader mental health field, ethical practices are highly focused on adults and require modification when working with children. However, there is information on common ethical issues with children not presented in codes. Some of those resources are listed below along with the website for the organization. Consider the following:

- American Association for Marriage and Family Therapists (2015): https://aamft.org/
- National Association of Social Workers (2021): https://www.socialworkers.org/
- American Psychological Association (2017): https://www.apa.org/
- American Psychiatric Association (2019): https://www.psychiatry.org/
- American Counseling Association (2014): https://www.counseling.org/

DOI: 10.4324/9781003189701-7

Group-specific Guidelines:

- The American Group Psychotherapy Association/International Board for Certification of Group Psychotherapists (2002): https://www.agpa.org/
- The International Association for Group Psychotherapy and Group Processes (2009): https://www.iagp.com/
- Barlow, S. H. (2013). *Specialty competencies in group psychology.* Oxford University Press. https://doi.org/10.1093/med:psych/9780195388558.001.0001
- Barlow, S., Burlingame, G.M., Greene, L.R., Joyce, A., Kaklauskas, F., Kinley, J., Klein, R.H., Kobos, J.C., Leszcz, M., MacNair-Semands, R., Paquin, J.D., Tasca, G.A., Whittingham, M., & Feirman, D. (2015). *Evidence-based practice in group psychotherapy. American Group Psychotherapy.* http://www.agpa.org/home/practice-resources/evidence-based-practice-in-group-psychotherapy
- Bernard, H., Burlingame, G., Flores, P., Greene, L., Joyce, A., Kobos, J. C., Leszcz, M., MacNair-Semands, R. R., Piper, W. E., Slocum McEneaney, A. M., Feirman, D. (2008). Clinical practice guidelines for group psychotherapy. *International Journal of Group Psychotherapy*, 58(4), 455–542. https://doi.org/10.1521/ijgp.2008.58.4.455
- Brabender, V., & MacNair-Semands, R. (2022). *The ethics in group psychotherapy: Principles and practical strategies.* New York: Routledge.
- Burlingame, G.M., Strauss, B., Joyce, A., MacNair-Semands, R., MacKenzie, K.R., Ogrodniczuk, J., & Taylor, S. (2006). *CORE Battery—Revised: An Assessment Tool Kit for Promoting Optimal Group Selection, Process and Outcome.* American Group Psychotherapy Association.
- Leszcz, M. (2018). The Evidence-Based Group Psychotherapist. *Psychoanalytic Inquiry*, 38, 285–298. https://doi.org/10.1080/07351690.2018.1444853
- Leszcz, M., & Kobos, J. C. (2008). Evidence-based group psychotherapy: Using AGPA's practice guidelines to enhance clinical effectiveness. *Journal of Clinical Psychology*, 64: 1238–1260. https://doi.org/10.1002/jclp.20531

Child-Specific Resources:

- American Academy of Child and Adolescent Psychiatry (2010): https://www.aacap.org/
- Sartor, T.A., McHenry, B., & McHenry, J. (Eds.). (2016). Ethical and Legal Issues in Counseling Children and Adolescents (1st ed.). Routledge. https://doi.org/10.4324/9781315660714

Telepsychology:

- American Psychological Association. (2013). Guidelines for the practice of telepsychology. https://www.apa.org/practice/guidelines/telepsychology

Many of the group resources list above provide important information about the competencies movement which seeks to guide clinicians by combining scientific literature and consensus and define group treatment as a stand-alone practice (as opposed to secondary to individual therapy). A better picture of evidence-based group practice incorporates flexibility, clinical experiences, empirically supported treatments and practice guidelines. Ethical care inherently involves seeking best practices for a given treatment. Group therapy therefore requires additional information, training and/or supervision for clinicians to provide evidence-based care. The American Group Psychotherapy Association (AGPA) offers a Certified Group Psychotherapy (CGP) certification which helps clinicians receive further training specifically in group treatment.

In conjunction with the practice guidelines and ethical principles outlined in the aforementioned core principle codes, therapists must also adhere to local, state and federal laws regarding treatment. Generally speaking, laws supersede ethics codes while the two commonly go hand-in-hand. Mental health laws are designed to ensure that qualified individuals are making treatment decisions. It is imperative clinicians understand the laws relevant to their field to ensure the highest quality of care for clients and to maintain licensure requirements. For a full list of relevant federal laws in the United States, visit https://www.usa.gov/laws-and-regs.

Working with children, legal and ethical standards are critically important in regard to mandatory reporting laws for abuse and neglect. Most therapists have made or will make a call to local authorities, Child Protective Services (CPS), or Adult Protective Services (APS). **Knowing the mandatory laws regarding CPS and APS are imperative in child group therapy** as children may talk candidly about abuse or neglect experiences during group which require a report. Such circumstances are unfortunately unavoidable. Knowing the nuances of relevant reporting laws in your state and country ensures the safety of child clients. For example, a child in group might reveal witnessing physical violence between caregivers. In the United States, state laws differ on reporting intimate partner violence: Some mandate a report with known injuries, others require reporting only if partners are married, while many states do not require reporting if the child is the client (as opposed to the caregiver). Clinicians must familiarize themselves with the individual reporting laws of the state in which they practice.

Laws often work together fluidly with the cultural morality upon which ethical principles are founded. **Morality encompasses the overarching frameworks used by the individual in making ethical decisions about what they consider to be right or wrong**. Morality is dependent on context, culture and the individual(s) making the decision.

Most ethical principles in mental health treatment are founded upon five basic, aspirational principles:

1 **Beneficence and Non-maleficence**: Promoting well-being and striving to do no harm;
2 **Fidelity**: Faithful follow-through of promises made to service recipients;
3 **Integrity**: Honest, transparent practice;
4 **Justice**: Equitable treatment of clients regardless of identity;
5 **Respect/Autonomy**: Respect for the client's right to self-direction within and outside of treatment.

Guiding principles such as these are the blueprints for the broader codes of ethics spanning therapy. At base, the point is to provide client care which is focused on their well-being and honestly puts forth change in service of the client rather than therapist needs.

Ethical Decision-Making

Thomas Hurster in Haen and Aronson (2017) provides a concise set of common steps seen across contemporary decision-making models:

1   "Assessment of the problem situation and ethical dimensions within the context in which it occurs.
2   Description and definition of the potential ethical conflict(s).
3   Application of professional codes and relevant legal statutes; outside consultation should be considered.
4   Development of alternative responses to the situation.
5   Applying ethical principles, an assessment is made of the consequences of alternative responses.
6   Implementation of the selected course of action.
7   Evaluation of the action taken, which will likely be ongoing." (p. 68)

Hurster's thoughtful consideration of various decision-making models encourages the sustained practices of consultation with professionals, legal statutes and professional ethical standards to inform ongoing ethical practice. Consider Johnson (2020) and Francis (2015) who offer public theses comparing decision-making models for mental health professionals. Ultimately, having a clearly defined method to identify ethical dilemmas and make informed decisions prevents lapses in judgment. Beyond the overarching moral principles guiding psychotherapy as a field, virtue- or morality-based decision-making models exist to clarify how to make sound ethical decisions on a personal level. Hurster discusses the importance of virtue ethics, or "the character traits, values, and ideas of the group therapist." (p. 67) Virtue-based ethics differs from principal-based ethics since they focus on the therapist's individual values and their interpersonal connection to the group at large. Reflecting on individual moral values and how they relate to the changing landscape of youth subcultures is an aspect of clinician self-awareness worthy of consistent attention.

Exercise

Violent video games are a topic of considerable debate among parents and professionals. At what point should children be allowed to watch or play violent media and what impact does it have on their developing brains and selves? While the answer to that question is complex and beyond the scope of this chapter, suffice to say the issue is a moral one because it ultimately entails an assessment of what is in the interest of the child. Some parents say children should not be allowed to play violent video games, or video games at all, while others would say the impact is negligible and children should be allowed to watch or play violent media at a young age. Varied responses such as these are rooted in moral judgment tied to culture and context. Child clinicians are often asked to comment on screen time and specific content children view.

In a situation like this, what would you recommend to parents? From where does that decision stem? What would you consider to be your moral foundations? Where did you learn right/wrong and what are the cultural underpinnings to your "moral compass"? What does it mean to be an ethical group practitioner with children? How would you blend both your moral values and the values of your client to make an informed recommendation?

Think about the ways in which you make ethical decisions. How do you reflect on them and who do you rely on as an "ethics buddy," or another professional with whom you consult about ethical dilemmas? How do you stay up-to-date on current research, theory and practice in groups with children?

Confidentiality

Trust is the building block of any therapeutic relationship. Without trust, any working alliance is unlikely to succeed or create change. Confidentiality in child groups requires an idiosyncratic application of development and knowledge of client's individual systems. As a starting point, clinicians must maneuver client disclosure and relationship-building with not just the child but important others who are part of the treatment process such as staff, caregivers and other group members. **Confidentiality remains one of the most challenging aspects of ethics with children, since navigating what to tell caregivers about treatment has both legal and ethical implications** (Sori & Hecker, 2015). This is inherently magnified in the group setting where confidentiality cannot be guaranteed between participants. Children who do not understand the importance of confidentiality will also not fully understand the impact that breaches can have on individuals and the treatment process.

Children, regardless of setting, bring issues of abuse, neglect, social media use, bullying and even drug use into sessions. Furthermore, children are often unaware of the impact of breaching confidentiality, as they are "open books" about their own lives. Child clinicians must therefore be comfortable with navigating confidentiality and its limits. Because of children's honest, "open-book" approach, what one child says in group may also be shared with that child's caregivers, peers, teachers or other important others. Setting plays an important role here. Settings for group therapy with children include:

- Schools
- Private Practice
- Inpatient Hospitals
- Residential Facilities
- Community Mental Health Centers
- Religious Centers
- Intensive Outpatient Units
- Juvenile Detention Centers

Within each of these settings, confidentiality has a different emphasis and meaning. For example, in a residential treatment facility or school, member-to-member confidentiality is typically paramount as opposed to private practice where client-caregiver confidentiality often takes priority. Member-to-member disclosures are generally less important in private practice because there is typically less overlap between social circles. Clients only see each other when they attend group sessions. In settings like residential facilities or rural communities where clients are frequently interacting with each other outside of group, confidentiality becomes a tricky dynamic. The more embedded the group is in a system in which the group members populate (such as a school or residential program), the more likely that confidentiality will be breached due to overlapping roles and relationships. In those systems, external boundaries are necessary to encourage active and honest participation in groups. If child clients are afraid peers will use their intimate information outside of group, what is their motivation for participating in group interventions? In a juvenile detention center, disclosures during a group session could realistically be used to promote violence or bullying against the disclosing member.

In a small, rural community mental health center where the clients and caregivers also know each other well, child clients might share group experiences with caregivers which could lead to unintentional conflict. In outpatient settings where clients share a broader community such as a school or place of worship, client disclosures can greatly impact their functioning in that community. If a trans child discloses their gender identity inside a known anti-trans religious community group, that child might be ostracized within the broader community if that information is shared outside of group. The trans client might not be allowed to have play dates with friends or participate in social activities as a direct result of the disclosure.

Technology brings a completely separate layer for confidentiality. Without realizing it, clients can break confidentiality by sharing their user location on social media, friending group members via video games, or taking a photo of another group member while in the waiting room. The ubiquitous accessibility the internet and cell phones/tablets provide also creates a simple method to inadvertently share protected information. All of these topics must be discussed with child group members and caregivers, sometimes as the unique incidents present themselves, so that privacy may be maintained.

The above examples illustrate the importance of confidentiality and what can happen should clinicians not work to ensure it as much as they can. While simplistic in theory, confidentiality in groups is a tricky concept which demands clinician forethought and clear boundaries.

Consider an inpatient group of children ages 9–13 at a long-term residential treatment center focusing on oppositional and conduct disorder clients. During a group session, one of the members, Grayson, directly microassaulted another group member, Alejandro, using a racial epithet. This led to a physical fight between the two boys which escalated quickly and Grayson was sent to the Emergency Room after being knocked unconscious. Think about all the different layers of confidentiality in this scenario. How do you protect Alejandro's identity when sharing the incident with staff at the treatment center? What about professionals in the Emergency Room? How would you share this incident with both of their families or caregivers and to what extent would you share details of the event itself? How would you process this in the group at the residential setting when all of the clients have to continue to work, learn and live together?

Confidentiality breaches are probable when keeping in mind children's innate lack of impulse control and developing knowledge of abstract concepts such as information privacy. Each relationship within child groups creates another "layer" of which child group clinicians must monitor. Each "layer" presents another opportunity for confidentiality to be breached, often unintentionally. Here are several examples of the multiple "layers" of confidentiality in child groups:

- Child-child
- Child-caregiver
- Child-therapist
- Therapist-caregiver
- Therapist-teacher
- Therapist-staff (such as at a residential or correctional facility)
- Client-social media
- Therapist-social media

These are just a few examples. Settings such as forensic units have additional layers of complexity while some such as private practice have fewer. **Child group therapists need to consider the complexities involved given the likelihood breaches in confidentiality will occur in group settings**. The many layers of confidentiality of groups make it tough to ethically provide treatment without considerable planning, preparation and intervention.

While many children might find the subject boring, firm boundaries and expectations about confidentiality during intakes or initial group sessions can be highly effective in building trusting environments. In structured environments, this may also include delineating what happens should clients break confidentiality outside of group. **Strong, concrete boundaries about confidentiality allow for increased emotional safety**. By overlapping child development onto the subject of confidentiality, therapists can find creative ways to make confidentiality fun. Playing a game of "telephone," role-playing basic feelings about confidentiality breaches and visual representations are all examples. Without explicit instruction, children are more likely than not to accidentally share confidential information.

Using the example above between Grayson and Alejandro, imagine that afternoon a member of the same group, Steven, posted about the fight on all of his social media accounts revealing the names of those involved. Steven detailed specifically what happened, what Grayson said and how Alejandro "mopped the floor with him with a chair." How would you manage Steven's posts? How would you talk to Steven about it? What about the rest of the group, including Grayson and Alejandro?

Two areas of confidentiality are exceptionally difficult to handle with children: Social media use and caregivers. Once something like Steven's posts are online, damage can be done surprisingly quickly. The average age of getting a smartphone is 10 and the average age of starting at least one social media account is 11 (Brigham, 2018). However, children are often incapable of understanding the risks of social media to themselves and others while able to access content which may be difficult for their developing minds to appropriately process. Inevitably, children end up creating content on social media which can have far-reaching effects. Maintaining confidentiality in a social media world becomes a daunting task when child group members may be tempted to share identifying information without realizing the potential harm.

Caregiver-client confidentiality remains another tricky balance to navigate when working with children. In the example above, Grayson's parents will need to be notified of the incident without sharing Alejandro's information. However, should they choose to press charges, the residential treatment facility may have no option but to provide Alejandro's confidential information. It is easy to see the cascade that follows one incident. Though it varies based on state laws, primary caregivers have legal access to child records and content of therapy sessions. This presents several unique quandaries for the child group clinician: How can you maintain confidentiality within group membership, knowing that children might tell caregivers about private disclosures and what are the limits to confidentiality between children and caregivers?

Grayson's parents are friends with other caregivers they met throughout the residential treatment process. Through the caregiver grapevine, they were able to see Steven's Facebook post about the fight. The staff at the residential treatment center were busy handling the event internally and ensuring Grayson's physical health and had not yet reached out to his parents. Grayson's parents started packing to go visit Grayson at the hospital and are furiously calling the treatment center. If this was your group, how would you handle speaking to them?

While caregivers are legally entitled to the content of sessions, children are ethically owed confidentiality should they not wish to share certain content with caregivers. Navigating what to tell caregivers, in addition to when confidentiality needs to be broken to local law enforcement or Child Protective Services, is a unique challenge within child groups. Explicitly talking about barriers to confidentiality with both children and caregivers can be an effective way to navigate these situations. This includes talking about exactly what will or will not be shared with caregivers or staff to set a containing boundary around the group. A boundary in this sense is an agreement, either formal or informal, with client and caregivers about what will and will not be shared from group sessions. Explicitly labeling the information to be given allows a concrete framework for children. Since confidentiality in groups cannot be guaranteed in the same way it can be within one-on-one therapeutic relationships, communication is key. Directly labeling the types of information shared between leaders and caregivers at the beginning of a client's group treatment helps all parties involved to know limits to confidentiality. This creates a foundation for clients to disclose personal information during group sessions. Group leaders can then build on this foundation by processing confidentiality and lapses in it during the life of the group.

Confidentiality is one of the most challenging ethical aspects of child groups due to the multiple layers of boundaries. So how does a child clinician set limits to promote sharing and prevent harm as much as possible? **A thoughtful consideration of how to intentionally address them within your practice setting can prevent many issues**.

Informed consent is an incredibly important part of all therapeutic services, especially group. Informed consent ultimately sets the stage for confidentiality in groups by delineating the limits to sharing information from group sessions with outsiders along with the risks and benefits of treatment. Informed consent provides a written avenue to help children and caregivers understand the point and limits of confidentiality. The highly contextual nature of settings means how and when to discuss and reinforce disclosure boundaries are unique to each group. Confidentiality must be discussed during any pre-group interviews and during the first group session to establish a foundation.

A developmental strategy to talk about this complex subject is to use child egocentrism to your advantage. Simply put, asking children what they would want shared outside of group using concrete examples can be highly effective. You might encourage children to only talk about broad topics (the content) as opposed to what individual members said (the process). The same goes for using the names of individual members with adults outside of group. Specific, concrete guidelines such as encouraging children to talk about their specific experiences as opposed to the names or actions of other group members plays to the concrete thinking of childhood. That way when asked what was discussed during sessions, it is less about the individual members and more about the content provided by leaders, goals or interventions. Strategies such as "sharing rules," or listing limits to confidentiality during group sessions in kid-friendly language, are ways to make this concrete subject considerably more kid-friendly.

Consider a 12-year-old presenting for services due to a major depressive episode. They may not want other members' caregivers to know. During the intake session, making this directly relevant to the client can illustrate the importance of confidentiality. Instead of depicting situations from other members and whether to share those situations outside of group, create an example for this specific member to use their egocentrism and personalize the point. You might say something along the lines of "Confidentiality can be tough to get sometimes. In group we will be working to help you feel better about yourself. We might practice being positive, flexible, or pushing back against nasty thoughts in our heads. If you talked about feeling sad because of being bullied at school for your haircut, would you want other people to share that with their families? (Client nods 'no') I wouldn't either. Those are the kind of situations to keep in group. It's not that you can't share things that happen in group with your family. You absolutely can. While your information and experience are your own, we ask that you keep specific examples like that or details about the other people in group private, just like you would want your details to be kept private. When in doubt, imagine how you would feel if somebody shared with their family what you are about to tell yours. Put yourself in their shoes. If you would feel uncomfortable, that's a good sign to not share!"

As individual circumstances arise, expectations surrounding confidentiality in group can be reinforced to remind child clients what they should and should not say about group sessions. After discussing a serious topic with a lot of shared information, you could remind clients that the individual disclosures remain in group. **The child group therapist can attend to potential breaches in the here-and-now by simply reminding the group about confidentiality rules**. Reinforcing expectations about confidentiality is a simple way to promote this boundary. As is often the case, intentionality is key. The more you think through potential barriers and breaches ahead of time, the more you prepare for them in your clinical practice.

Exercise

One of your outpatient groups is for children five to eight years old. One of your group members comes in and tells you his father got angry this week and yelled at him for playing video games when he was supposed to be eating dinner with the family. There is no known history of abuse within the family. The group member does not seem upset by the situation and is calm when talking about it.

Several weeks later, the same child talks about his father yelling at him again, this time with an increased level of intensity. The child becomes upset while talking about it. When pressed for further information, the child shuts down and refuses to speak. The same is true outside of session.

The week after that incident, the same child says his father came into his room, yelled at him and forcefully pulled him away from his video games, leaving a handprint of bruises on his arm. The client is notably upset and cries when talking about it, pleading with the group therapist to not tell his parents.

Think about the many ways and points in time from this scenario in which one might intervene.

At what point would you break confidentiality? Why? And to whom? How would you respond to this child during group?

In this case, the bare minimum includes notifying Child Protective Services after the last disclosure as the child is overtly harmed. Situations such as this one are unfortunately commonplace for child clinicians. Two ethical recommendations include:

- Having a peer consultation group or an ethics "buddy" to help with navigating state/local/federal laws and ethics applied to specific scenarios; and
- Create a "decision tree" while identifying possible steps and the impact it may have on the child and their family/caregiver system.

Children are often coached into not talking about certain subjects or experiences, just like they are encouraged for bringing in significant situations into group. Decision trees and ethics groups/buddies provide sounding boards while navigating the context-specific ethical decisions within child treatment.

Logistical and Clinical Ethics for Child Groups

Many ethical dilemmas arise from simple logistical concerns not addressed during group formation, forming or conclusion. **All stages of group planning and preparation must include forethought of ethical concerns to prevent ethical or legal predicaments**. Common solutions involve dutiful preparation, effective communication and transparency which are evident in the dilemmas below. With a little foresight and practice-specific examination, many violations can be avoided!

Advertising and Recruitment

The advertising, marketing, recruitment of group members, group composition, note-taking and responsibilities of the leader(s) are often-neglected aspects of ethical group preparation, and all of them happen prior to scheduling an intake. Ethical care starts before clients even enter the door!

Advertising for psychological services may feel uncomfortable for many clinicians. Many therapists enter the field with the purpose of helping others and do not have a background in marketing or business. Advertising has legal and ethical implications as it communicates to the public and other professionals basic facts about the group. Careful consideration of group composition and ideal clients creates a method for communication with others about the specific group you propose. As with advertising any service, state and federal laws govern what can and cannot be said about groups. Clinicians knowingly misleading the public can cause significant harm, thus state and federal laws control the depiction of advertisements. **All advertising materials must accurately depict the purpose of the group, the credentials of the service provider and refrain from guaranteed statements about therapeutic impact**. While this might sound common sense, it is easy to see how misguided clinicians could inadvertently misrepresent themselves or their services. Even trickier, in therapy we cannot rely on client testimonials without significant attention related to informed consent. When in doubt, always consult with a colleague with some experience or expertise in the area.

Recruiting appropriate members for a child group is considerably more difficult than it sounds, especially when seeking referrals from professionals outside of child mental health. Other professionals may not consider all of the factors influencing goodness of fit in a specific group and become irritated when their referral is not accepted. Before a group even begins, clinicians must carefully consider who would make a reasonably good fit for the intended group and find ways to communicate a "client prototype" with referral sources.

Paperwork and Record-Keeping

Another seemingly simple but important task is record-keeping. Note-taking is a surprisingly demanding aspect of any clinical role but especially for groups considering the sheer volume of records to be completed. Each state has basic but mandatory requirements for session records. While second nature to many clinicians and electronic medical record systems, balancing what to include in notes and how to write about group processes is often left to on-the-job training and supervision. **Group leader(s) must consider who will be responsible for notes, when they can be anticipated to be finished and how to talk about group processes in notes without sharing the identifying information of other group members**. This represents a surprisingly big feat for novel group clinicians. Simple communication about clinical notes can be enough to prevent a more serious ethical lapse throughout the life of a group.

The formality of completing forms at the start of a professional relationship also sets the parameters for treatment. It helps clients know what to expect, limits to the therapeutic relationship such as expected outcomes and confidentiality, what treatment is like and placement policies for details like attendance and cost. While it may be tedious at times, paperwork is essential to quality care. Working with children, clinicians must know how, what and with whom to communicate. Paperwork and orientation to the group process are ethical considerations to make before clients start. **Paperwork including role induction, limits to confidentiality and informed consent are incredibly important to ethical care**. Clients coming into a group, especially children, may have no experience with group therapy. Role induction involves talking about the processes of the group, potential content, and expectations for the client during sessions. This process provides clarity for children who may be nervous or oppositional about starting in a group. In addition to role induction, clients need a basic overview of confidentiality, how to ensure it between group members and with caregivers or staff and informed consent about group therapy services. All of the essential intake paperwork needs to be tailored to group sessions and provided in a child-friendly way to both clients and any caregivers who ultimately have access to medical records. This may include creating specific guidelines or paperwork for group clients which are separate from individual therapy clients. **Intake paperwork and role inductions orient both client and caregivers to the process of group therapy before they start in a group**.

Extra-group Communication and Relationships in Child Groups

Oftentimes clinicians must provide the same information to both children and care providers simultaneously which makes certain aspects of establishing care challenging to communicate. Informed consent is particularly tricky when it comes to children and in complex settings such as residential treatment facilities. In an outpatient setting, informed consent typically revolves around the content discussed in group, the legal limits to confidentiality (suicidal and homicidal intent) and what will or will not be communicated to caregivers. However, the waters are murkier in residential settings or schools where confidentiality cannot be guaranteed and has broader implications. Participants need to be informed of the potential risks and benefits of being in group with people whom they live with or have multiple relationships. Multiple relationships range from acquaintances to personal, familial, romantic or antagonistic relationships between clients. Sometimes, in settings such as schools, community mental health centers or outpatient practices, members have a clear relationship they bring into a group. Those relationships can interfere with the members' abilities to participate. Due to the legal limits of confidentiality, clinicians often do not know of pre-existing relationships between group members.

Imagine you are leading a group for children with mood disorders ages 10–13 at a local school. Due to the pandemic, the school is reporting high levels of mood and behavioral disruptions. You are about to interview the seventh member, Jeremy, for this group, a child known throughout the school because of his highly disruptive behavior. Given your work as a clinician in the school, you routinely see the social exclusion resulting from Jeremy's behavioral outbursts. Jeremy has "meltdowns" which can last upwards of an hour and happen multiple times per week. Several of the other members you interviewed for joining the group spontaneously identified disliking Jeremy due to his outbursts. Do you allow him in your group? What are the risks and benefits for including Jeremy?

The above scenario is incredibly common. Pre-group screenings are helpful tools which prevent groups failing from lack of cohesion or prior relationships. Such multiple relationships are not always bad but have the potential to disrupt group processes. They are often assessed at the beginning of the therapeutic relationship to prevent major issues. In an outpatient setting, clients who attend the same grade at the same school are likely to be placed in separate groups to prevent their existing relationship from impacting group processes. Outside of the very obvious boundaries of multiple relationships (not having siblings in the same group, for example) more nuanced distinctions must be considered. In a school setting, it is common to have friends or classmates in group together. Such multiple relationships need to be carefully considered in terms of their impact on the group. If two best friends attend the same group, it can negatively impact group processes and dampen the client's individual growth. **While not inherently bad and at times unavoidable, multiple relationships are best considered during the beginning phase of a group so clinicians and**

members can decide how to handle them. If they are unavoidable, conversations during the initial phase can ease children's minds. Simply talking about how to handle the relationship and anything which happens outside of sessions models appropriate boundaries and communication. Children are wonderfully creative with their solutions with how to greet a fellow group member should they see each other in a shared setting like school. Children respond to basic, concrete boundaries which allow them to solve the issue in a way which feels appropriate to them, such as acknowledging each other at school but not speaking about group content. Sometimes the two group members even prepare a response to their friends if asked how the two know each other!

During a group session, you notice two members have become close. They have many inside jokes which are clearly from contact outside of group sessions. They laugh frequently and make asides to one another. The following session, you notice the same two members appear to be distant. They make subtle insults towards each other and mention the other is a bad friend. What missing information would you need to make an informed decision regarding these two members' outside contact? In what ways would the missing information change your clinical judgment about this scenario? What are your steps in resolving this conflict?

The details from this clinical vignette were purposefully absent. Setting, client presentation, nature of the outside contact and the impact it has on the working group (among other variables) are all critical components in how to handle a situation involving clients contacting each other outside of group treatment. Whatever the context, extra-group contact such as this one must be discussed within the confines of the group to ensure continued group safety.

Therapist Dual Roles

If a therapist and client have another existing relationship, this is referred to as a dual relationship. While not always iatrogenic, any dual relationship must be considered carefully. A common example is a clinician who chooses to see group clients for individual therapy. Like all potential dual relationships between clinician and client, clients need to know how the two might impact each other. Some schools of thought consider seeing a client for both individual and group therapy simultaneously to be unethical. However, over the years, this viewpoint has shifted to a more client-driven viewpoint which highlights the potential advantages of this dual relationship (Türk, 2019).

Communication provides an effective way to manage this particular dual relationship. Clinicians can seek permission to share content from an individual session or bring up a topic which is a focus of individual treatment but not group treatment. In other words, it is better to over-communicate and seek permission from clients rather than accidentally share private content from an individual session during group.

In smaller communities, sometimes dual roles are unavoidable. If a clinician is the sole group provider for children in their town, children of their friends or classmates of their own children may seek services. Individual ethical codes address dual roles and the moral parameters governing them, but suffice to say that when avoidable, dual roles are best left separate.

Group Composition: Balancing the Needs of the Group vs. the Needs of the Individual

Group composition is an integral task for starting any group. **Even at an early stage, leaders must balance the needs of the group with the needs of the individual**. In some settings, leaders do not choose the members while in others they have complete autonomy.

In settings where control is an option, inclusion/exclusion criteria can be incredibly helpful in deciding who would be good members for a particular group while also communicating with referral sources about appropriate clients.

Balancing the needs of the group with the needs of the individual can provide a tricky ethical dilemma. Group composition is part of the nuts-and-bolts which drives cohesion. Refining composition by using inclusion/exclusion criteria for the group's goals and following through with whether or not to allow certain members to participate impacts group outcomes. The same is true for early stages where members may regularly confront each other and authority. The "storming" phase brings out the dilemma of balance: When does the need of one individual member take precedence over the group as a whole? Deciding when one takes priority takes considerable clinical judgment. One member may completely sabotage a group if leaders do not prioritize the health of the group as a whole.

Due to restraints on your time and push from the school (despite your clinical judgment), Jeremy joined your group. Things have gone smoother than expected until the third session where Jeremy has one of his "meltdowns." He did not want to leave the group to go back to class and 15 minutes prior to the end of the group started yelling and insulting you and the other members. This does not abate for the remainder of the session and only escalates, with Jeremy picking up his chair and throwing it across the room, narrowly missing two other members. The other members are visibly scared by Jeremy's escalation. It is now time for the group to conclude so that children can go home for the day. What do you do in the moment? How do you handle the situation specifically related to the other group members and their physical/emotional safety? How do you handle the situation systemically with the school, caregivers or significant others?

In the example above, the leader is placed in a situation where they must consider the individual (Jeremy) having a meltdown or the success of the group as a whole. The impacts are evident in the members' frightened responses to Jeremy's behavior. If this repeatedly happens, the group is likely to lack a healing impact and instead have a damaging effect on the rest of the members. In such situations, it is the responsibility of the leader(s) to advocate for the group as a whole despite the needs of one of the members.

Co-Leader Considerations

In groups using a co-leadership model, how is the work split? Equitable co-leadership may not seem like a common ethical dilemma, but co-leadership issues can easily derail the therapeutic benefit of group sessions. In practice with children, it is helpful to articulate who will be responsible for what role either in a single group session or the length of the group. It is best to do so at the outset of the group, so there are clear expectations between leaders. For example, one group leader might do all of the group intakes while the other is responsible for group session notes. Dividing up the work of the group, including leadership roles such as putting one leader in charge of content while the other is in charge of process, can help the group run smoothly and facilitate positive communication.

How will conflict between group leaders be handled? Conflict between co-leaders as group cohesion develops is often missed as a potential dilemma which can be ruinous to child groups. How do you handle when a co-leader isn't performing their duties or there is a personality conflict? During the life of a group, conflict is bound to happen between co-leaders.

You and your co-leader have been working together for three years running an inpatient group at a local hospital. Your co-leader recently divorced and for several weeks has been showing up late, disheveled and quiet. At times, you suspect they are hungover or still drunk. One time, they fell asleep during a session. In this group, you are responsible for planning the content while your co-leader does the notes. Your supervisor tells you that the notes from this group have not been completed in over a month. What are your decision-making steps to resolve this conflict?

As is much of the case in ethical dilemmas with other professionals, the starting point is addressing the concerns directly with the clinician. Should this not successfully resolve the conflict, other measures may need to be taken to prevent harm to clients. Larger agencies, hospitals and community mental health hospitals should have procedures and policies which clinicians can use to guide conflict situations with co-leaders. Steps might include reprimands, removal from the group as a co-leader or, in particularly egregious situations, termination.

Therapist Stress and Burn-out

Leading child groups is no easy feat. Difficult caseloads, paperwork, systemic issues and personal factors can lead to stress and burn-out. 21–61% of mental health clinicians show signs of burn-out (Morse et al., 2012). It is easy to see how emotional fatigue and workplace stress can negatively impact therapist job performance, especially with children. The vulnerable nature of children and the shocking heaviness of child therapy can create ethical dilemmas for even the most talented clinicians. Child group clinicians have to harness and develop change within a chaotic environment which consumes considerable emotional energy. Outside of the emotional energy expended during child groups, there is additional physical energy used in play interventions. All of this is to say child groups require significant internal resources which can lead to burn-out during times of clinician stress. Without careful observation and management, burn-out can lead to negative therapy outcomes and physical ailments amongst practitioners (Kim et al., 2011).

Clinician self-care is touted as an integral part of ethical care, yet there is surprisingly little guidance on how to handle the emotional fatigue that comes with therapy. Mental health therapists are containers for the emotions of others yet have to figure out how to let go of that emotional energy in a way which is productive and not self-destructive. Fortunately, many therapeutic techniques used with clients are helpful in combating burn-out. For example, both problem-solving skills and mindfulness skills can be used to reduce clinician burn-out (Jergensen, 2017; Somoray et al., 2017). It is therefore paramount for clinicians to engage in meaningful forms of self-care which facilitate emotional boundaries from clinical work.

Self-care holds a different meaning for each person. Part of the reason clinician self-care is so amorphous is because of the subjective nature of self-care; people "recharge" their emotional batteries in unique ways. Regardless of the ways in which stress is reduced, intentional self-care practice can reduce stress and burn-out.

The various systems in which therapists operate can also impact burn-out. In addition to personal skills, workplace support and value can help reduce burn-out on a systemic level (Viehl et al., 2017). In supportive systems where work and workers alike are valued, the culture of burn-out can shift.

Take a moment to reflect on your self-care routines and strategies. How do you know when you need to engage in self-care? How do you know if your self-care strategy works? What are three things you do as an individual to let go of the emotional heaviness of psychotherapy? What are two things you would consider adding as part of your self-care?

Suicidal Ideation in Child Groups

While death by suicide in children under 12 remains relatively rare, this number continues to rise with little information on mitigating factors (Ayer, 2020). According to the Center for

Disease Control (CDC), suicide is the eighth leading cause of death amongst children and the second leading cause of death amongst adolescents (Ayer, 2020; Ruch et al., 2021). Suicidal ideation brings a number of ethical considerations when present in child groups. As discussed previously when talking about informed consent, it is vital caregivers and children alike understand the risks and benefits of informed consent, especially as it relates to federal and state laws regarding client disclosure. Child group therapists must know whom to contact regarding suicidal ideation (relevant local resources and caregivers) and how to talk about limits of confidentiality in a developmentally appropriate manner. Informed consent is critically important to suicidal clients as it promotes autonomy, privacy, and respect for their treatment (Bernert & Roberts, 2012).

Like with individual therapy, clients must be able to both talk about suicidal ideation and know the limits to confidentiality should it need to be breached in favor of their physical safety. This brings a unique dynamic to child groups, where some children may express suicidal thoughts while others have no concept of it. The fears of suicide "contagion," where talking about suicide leads to other group members expressing or acting on thoughts of suicide, or "clusters," where suicide occurs very frequently around a singular person or point, are common. While both have research support, they remain largely unclear due to the number of complex factors which impact death by suicide (Walling, 2021). Research suggests that talking about suicide is ultimately more likely to reduce risk than create further harm (Dazzi et al., 2014). **Therefore, in child groups, assessing for, talking about and monitoring suicidal ideation is an important ethical task**.

Ruch et al. (2021) identify several themes from amongst the childhood death by suicide literature:

- Mental health and suicide-related concerns,
- Trauma,
- Family-related problems, and
- School or peer-related problems.

No factor is universally present in death by suicide. However, group therapists are ethically bound to observe their clients and presentation during group to decipher when and how to assess risk. This is especially true for clients with previously expressed suicidal ideation and considerable life stress. In these cases, monitoring suicidal thoughts and using clinical judgment to ensure safety is paramount. While the whole of suicide prevention literature is beyond the scope of this book, adequate and consistent assessment can help prevent suicidal actions.

Post-Group Ethical Considerations

The end of a group's life brings about unique ethical situations. Continuity of relationships and concluding treatment are two important scenarios to think about as a group moves towards termination. When a group concludes, particularly child groups, children may want to continue contact with other members. Group leaders therefore must consider what boundaries to suggest or encourage when a group ends. In some instances, children may want to become friends after a group ends or seek contact through social media, video games or play dates. Termination becomes an ethical consideration to ensure clients finish services as positively as possible.

As with many ethical considerations, forethought and communication are helpful allies. Children often present specifically for group treatment because of social disruptions as part of their diagnoses. If clinicians make decisions about the implications of friendships outside of group and whether to allow them as part of the group's life, then messages about termination and continuation of relationships are clear. Child clients differ from adult clients in their expectations of group therapy and in many outpatient settings use treatment as a way to build positive relationships. As conscientious as clinicians must be about multiple relationships and relationships formed in the group, there is equal importance on the positive impact of child clients continuing their relationships after group is finished or in some cases *during* group. While adult groups often have stricter boundaries, child clients are best served by carefully considering the potential risks *and benefits* of interpersonal boundaries as a group moves towards termination.

The end of the school year is near. Jeremy from the example above made considerable gains in treatment. He has a "frenemy" (youth term for somebody both a friend and an enemy with qualities of both) in group, Taj, with whom he wants to become better friends. Sometimes, Jeremy and Taj get along very well. At other times, they verbally fight or make mean "roast" comments to each other which are clearly hurtful. Jeremy really wants to be friends with Taj and talks about going to the skate park with him in the summer. Taj seems happy about the idea some days and unhappy other days. There are four more weeks left in the school year and the group. How do you handle this situation? Would you encourage further boundaries until the group is finished or encourage them to be friends? Would you openly discuss this during group? Why or why not?

There is no "right" or "wrong" answer to the social dilemma with Jeremy and Taj. Most ethical situations are shades of gray and you must rely on your own clinical judgment, with support from colleagues as sounding boards, to make the best decisions in the moment. When in doubt, ask a trusted colleague to ensure you are making a decision with the client's interest in mind!

Just like your decision about Jeremy and Taj is likely related to the phase of group, ethical termination is a tough consideration that is highly contextual. In acute hospitals, termination is handled by providers linking clients to outside services and there is little opportunity for closure during group. In long-term residential facilities or outpatient groups, termination takes on significant meaning. During the termination phase, child clients are given the opportunity to say a healthy goodbye and connect to any clinical recommendations. Ethical termination from group with children involves:

- Asking children their impressions of group and any growth;
- Rituals for saying goodbye and encouraging a healthy transition;
- Providing clients with clinical recommendations based on client growth; and
- Assessing treatment gains.

Saying goodbye to child clients, if done abruptly or not at all, directly feeds into narratives of abandonment or worthlessness. Ethical terminations challenge negative narratives by honoring the work of child clients during the group's life. Small rituals such as making a transition object during the final session, providing a certificate of graduation or simply talking about all of the changes in each member are within your power as a therapist. Making it a point to allow the group and each member to say goodbye is an important part of ethical practice!

Exercise

- From start to finish, what are some ethical practices you would like to bolster in your current groups? What about your future groups?
- How do you handle child clients and whether or not they should have contact with other group members outside of group?
- In what ways do you promote a healthy interpersonal goodbye?

Measurement-Based Care and Quality Assurance

There is a growing movement in psychotherapy which calls for clinicians to routinely use outcome measurements referred to as measurement-based care (Fortney et al., 2017). Measurement-based care emphasizes the use of various methods to monitor treatment progression with group therapy no exception. **Most leading authors in group and individual therapy recommend assessing outcomes at various intervals to ensure quality of care** (Corey et al., 2018; Sheppard, in Haen and Aronson, 2017; Shechtman, 2006). Outcomes provide a demonstrable impact of group. While it may not appear obvious at first, monitoring treatment effects are an ethical part of treatment. Outcomes are increasingly discussed in ethical standards. However, they are not enforced by law nor are they typically emphasized during training. Both client measurements and clinician reflection ensure quality of treatment, especially across long-running groups. Consider the following ways to measure outcomes:

- Client self-report/behavioral observation during sessions
- Caregiver/teacher/important adult report
- Behavior outcome measurements filled out by clients, such as repeated assessments of symptoms or behaviors (e.g. behavior rating scales or symptom checklists)
- Specific therapy outcome tools completed during sessions (e.g. Outcome Rating Scale/ Session Rating Scale)
- Clinician self-evaluation tools

Developmentally, children provide only limited information via self-report. Child reports can be used to guide feedback and when combined with a baseline provide one measure of progress. While this information is valuable, alternative measures supplement client self-report. Caregiver report, behavioral observations during group made by the therapist and assessment measures given to trusted adults all provide further objective evidence of treatment impact.

Pre-test and post-test measures at specific intervals during group treatment are simple and effective. During the clinical interview at the start of treatment, clinicians gather a baseline of client behaviors and goals. Adding in specific intervals, such as a feedback session or assessments with caregivers every 8–12 weeks during active treatment, can provide continued data to be compared to baseline and goals. Specific outcome measures used in individual therapy sessions are an alternative which offer session-by-session client self-report. However, since children can offer only limited data, other methods of evaluation are suggested to supplement self-report as discussed above.

Corey et al. (2018) also suggest using journaling, leadership rating tools and debriefing as methods for the therapist's self-evaluation. Therapist **self-evaluation tools help individual clinicians measure their own presence and interventions within each group**. Though simple in nature, the act of reflection on clinician behavior and client presentation ensures a continual monitoring inherently valuable in the change process. Sheppard, writing in Haen and Aronson (2017), talks about the value of a clinic- or practitioner-specific outcome measures which can be "…customized to the specific goals and needs of the individual group or program" (p. 48). Here are a few basic dos and don'ts for outcome measures:

- DO include children in their evaluation of group treatment
- DO find ways to use kid-friendly language so they may be involved
- DO gather data from multiple sources outside of group if possible
- DO inform children for what the data will be used
- DO store each individual member's records separately
- DO store all records of outcomes confidentially in the child's file
- DO NOT make references to identifying information of other group members in outcome measurements

- DO NOT share private information from group with outside professionals unless clinically necessary
- DO NOT promote unnecessary data collection, such as excessive assessments

Below is a sample of a child-friendly rating scale taken directly from the authors at our practice, Groupworks. Notice the kid-friendly language and use of simple faces to help children identify for themselves how they are progressing in treatment. Children fill out these forms every few months prior to feedback with caregivers about the child's response to group treatment. In general, Self-Esteem (SE), Self-Regulation (SR) and Interpersonal Skills (IS) are measured to track ongoing progress. Over time, clinicians can see changes and use the progress, or lack thereof, to guide goal-setting and interventions (Figure 7.1).

Think for a moment about your own use of outcome measures:

- What methods do you use to monitor client progress?
- What methods do you use to self-reflect on a group's life cycle and efficacy of leadership?
- Practically, what outcome measures or behavioral measurements might you consider incorporating into your child groups?

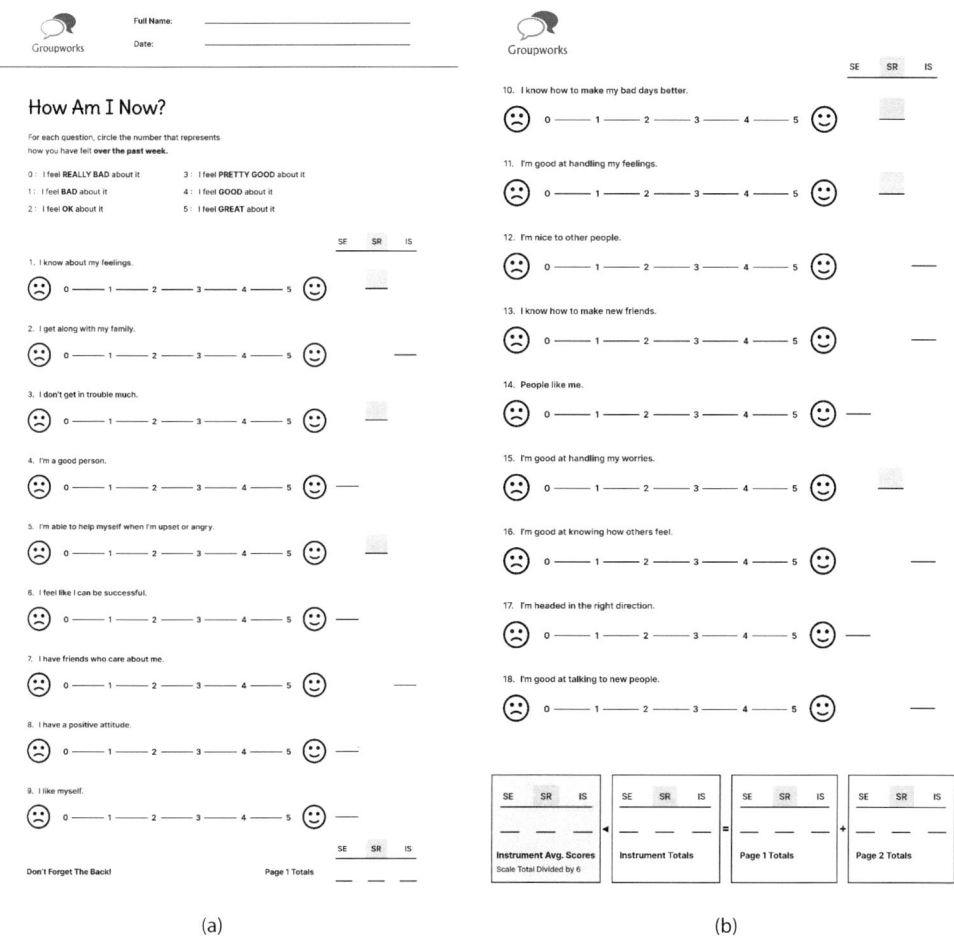

(a)   (b)

Figure 7.1 (a and b) How I am Now

Intersecting Diversity and Ethics

Practicing through a diversity framework is in every way an ethical one. Stemming from the basic concepts that are part of every ethical code, therapists strive to do no harm. Therefore, understanding culture and client identification within their culture and transgenerational history is a unique part of ethical care with children. **If we do not take time to understand our client's cultural identification and values, especially those different from our own and the majority culture, we run the risk of over-pathologizing, misunderstanding symptom presentations and providing iatrogenic care** (Wendt et al., 2015). If clinicians solely practice from dominant culture, they can miss the mark with interventions and unconsciously promote dominant culture values through therapeutic style. This is especially important noting the WEIRD (Western, educated, industrialized, rich, democratic) history of therapy from which definitions for pathology and "normalcy" are derived. In fact, norming samples are great examples which illustrate this point.

Many norming and research populations are taken from the same WEIRD convenience samples at universities which do not often compensate for the diversity of clients across the globe. In all reality, given the international use of popular psychological assessments, it would be close to impossible to represent all identities in one sample. So what happens when a client presenting for specific treatment or an assessment does not match the norming sample? There are no clear answers to this, but it is abundantly clear that if clinicians do not use a multicultural lens when providing treatment, they can cause harm to clients and further stigmatize therapy within those populations.

Often, clinicians are left to contextualize popular theories in order to meet client needs. As discussed during Chapter 3 on multicultural practice, modifications for therapy when done intentionally can be highly effective.

Decolonization of psychotherapeutic research, theories and interventions is a slowly developing turning point in behavioral science capable of transforming the field to be more globally inclusive (Adams et al., 2015; Gone, 2021; Goodman & Gorski, 2015; Mills, 2014). Practicing justice within the behavioral sciences necessitates removing the cultural assumptions of normative therapies in order to meet clients within their cultural frameworks. To ignore the cultures from which our clients exist and practice within would be to ignore their daily experiences.

The COVID-19 pandemic provides a clear example of the psychological impact of colonialism. Fueled by ignorance, conspiracy theories and political agendas, China was maligned and blamed for COVID-19. Chinese Americans and non-Chinese Asian-Americans were unjustly targeted as a result. During the pandemic, hate crimes targeting Asian-Americans rose dramatically, leading to significant levels of race-based trauma and trauma from interventions which may not be culturally sensitive (Litam, 2020). In California alone, the number of anti-Asian hate crimes rose 107% (California Department of Justice, 2020). Lack of culturally sensitive care shows how acting from a solely majority viewpoint pushes ideas about treatment or groups of people which can ultimately be iatrogenic. This illustrates the **clear importance of culturally attuned care as an ethical issue in all behavioral sciences**. Acting with integrity and justice toward our clients involves dismantling the structures which encourage power differentials and uphold discriminatory actions. Only then may equitable treatment be truly integrated into the practice of psychotherapy.

Inside and outside of therapy, children are owed the same level of respect provided to adults. It is easy to minimize the experiences of children and assume they do not understand issues of diversity. However, this is untrue. Groups bring unique opportunities for identity growth. The diversity within child groups can be teachable moments for clients.

Children are attuned to diversity and differences amongst group members. Differences allow for children to increase their sensitivity to and understanding of diversity. Taking the opportunities presented during group discussions and processes create a culturally sensitive environment.

To minimize microaggressions and children's subjective experiences is to negate their individual experiences. Children understand issues of diversity in the ways in which they are able, and those experiences are to be respected and processed as a healthy way to increase understanding of diversity. Treating children with dignity and respect can help undermine discriminatory systems by showing children their inherent worth.

Summary

The purpose of this chapter is to inform clinicians of the child-specific ethical issues relevant for effective practice and walk through scenarios to promote ethical decision-making. Despite the multitude of unique issues within child groups, creating and sustaining ethical practice is very attainable. Consider the ways in which you maintain an ethical practice and in doing so, how those ethical decisions positively impact the people you serve.

References

Adams, G., Dobles, I., Gomez, L. H., & Molina, L. E. (2015). Decolonizing psychological science (special thematic section). *Journal of Social and Political Psychology*, *3*(1). https://doi.org/10.5964/jspp.v3i1.564

American Academy of Child and Adolescent Psychiatry. (2010). AACAP Code of Ethical Principles. https://www.aacap.org/aacap/Member_Resources/Ethics/Foundation/AACAP_Code_of_Ethical_Principles.aspx

American Association for Marriage and Family Therapists. (2015). American Association for Marriage and Family Therapists Code of Ethics. https://www.aamft.org/Legal_Ethics/Code_of_Ethics.aspx

American Counseling Association. (2014). 2014 ACA code of ethics. https://www.counseling.org/docs/default-source/default-document-library/2014-code-of-ethics-finaladdress.pdf

American Group Psychotherapy Association. (2002). AGPA and IBCGP guidelines for ethics. https://www.agpa.org/home/practice-resources/ethics-in-group-therapy

American Psychological Association. (2013). Guidelines for the practice of telepsychology. https://www.apa.org/practice/guidelines/telepsychology

American Psychological Association. (2017). Ethical principles of psychologists and code of conduct (2002, amended effective June 1, 2010, and January 1, 2017). https://www.apa.org/ethics/code/

American Psychiatric Association. (2019). American Psychiatric Association's Principles of Medical Ethics with Annotations Especially Applicable to Psychiatry ("Principles"). https://www.psychiatry.org/psychiatrists/practice/ethics

Ayer, L., Colpe, L., Pearson, J., Rooney, M., & Murphy, E. (2020). Advancing research in child suicide: A call to action. *Journal of the American Academy of Child and Adolescent Psychiatry*, *59*(9), 1028–1035. https://doi.org/10.1016/j.jaac.2020.02.010

Barlow, S. H. (2013). *Specialty competencies in group psychology*. Oxford: Oxford University Press. https://doi.org/10.1093/med:psych/9780195388558.001.0001

Barlow, S., Burlingame, G. M., Greene, L. R., Joyce, A., Kaklauskas, F., Kinley, J., Klein, R. H., Kobos, J. C., Leszcz, M., MacNair-Semands, R., Paquin, J. D., Tasca, G. A., Whittingham, M., & Feirman, D. (2015). *Evidence-based practice in group psychotherapy. American Group Psychotherapy.* http://www.agpa.org/home/practice-resources/evidence-based-practice-in-group-psychotherapy

Bernard, H., Burlingame, G., Flores, P., Greene, L., Joyce, A., Kobos, J. C., Leszcz, M., MacNair-Semands, R. R., Piper, W. E., Slocum McEneaney, & A. M., Feirman, D. (2008). Clinical practice guidelines for group psychotherapy. *International Journal of Group Psychotherapy*, *58*(4), 455–542. https://doi.org/10.1521/ijgp.2008.58.4.455

Bernert, R. A., & Roberts, L. W. (2012). Ethics commentary: Suicide risk: Ethical considerations in the assessment and management of suicide risk. *Focus*, *10*(4), 467–472.

Brabender, V., & MacNair-Semands, R. (2022). *The ethics in group psychotherapy: Principles and practical strategies*. New York: Routledge.

Brigham, K. (2018, December). Facebook, Snapchat and TikTok have a massive underage user problem – here's why it matters. *CNBC*. https://www.cnbc.com/2018/12/21/what-age-is-appropriate-to-sign-up-for-social-media.html#:~:text=According%20to%20a%20report%20by, many%20lie%20about%20their%20age.

Burlingame, G. M., Strauss, B., Joyce, A., MacNair-Semands, R., MacKenzie, K. R., Ogrodniczuk, J., & Taylor, S. (2006). *CORE Battery—revised: An assessment tool kit for promoting optimal group selection, process and outcome*. New York: American Group Psychotherapy Association.

California Department of Justice, R. C. C. J. I. S. D. (2020). Anti-Asian Hate Crime Events During the COVID-19 Pandemic. Retrieved December 29, 2021. Retrieved from https://efaidnbmnnnib-pcajpcglclefindmkaj/viewer.html?pdfurl=https%3A%2F%2Foag.ca.gov%2Fsystem%2Ffiles%2Fme-dia%2Fanti-asian-hc-report.pdf&clen=614917

Corey, M. S., Corey, G., & Corey, C. (2018). *Groups: Process and practice*. Boston, MA: Cengage Learning.

Dazzi, T., Gribble, R., Wessely, S., & Fear, N. T. (2014). Does asking about suicide and related behaviours induce suicidal ideation? What is the evidence?. *Psychological Medicine*, *44*(16), 3361–3363. https://doi.org/10.1017/S0033291714001299

Fortney, J. C., Unützer, J., Wrenn, G., Pyne, J. M., Smith, G. R., Schoenbaum, M., & Harbin, H. T. (2017). A Tipping point for measurement-based care. *Psychiatric Services (Washington, D.C.)*, *68*(2), 179–188. https://doi.org/10.1176/appi.ps.201500439

Francis, P. C. (2015). A Review of Contemporary Ethical Decision-Making Models for Mental Health Professionals. Master's Thesis, Eastern Michigan University. ERIC.

Gone, J. P. (2021). Decolonization as methodological innovation in counseling psychology: Method, power, and process in reclaiming American Indian therapeutic traditions. *Journal of Counseling Psychology*, *68*(3), 259–270. https://doi.org/10.1037/cou0000500

Goodman, R. D., & Gorski, P. C. (Eds.). (2015). *Decolonizing "multicultural" counseling through social justice*. Cham: Springer Science + Business Media. https://doi.org/10.1007/978-1-4939-1283-4

Hurster, T. (2017) Ethically Informed Group Practice. In C. Haen, & S. Aronson (Eds.), *Handbook of child and adolescent group therapy: A practitioner's reference* (pp. 66–78). New York: Routledge.

International Association for Group Psychotherapy and Group Processes. (2009). IAGP's Ethical Guidelines and Professional standards for Group Psychotherapists. https://www.iagp.com/about/ethical-guidelines.htm

Jergensen, K. (2017). Practice what you preach: An exploration of DBT therapists personal skill utilization in burnout prevention. *Clinical Social Work Journal*. https://doi.org/10.1007/s10615-017-0633-6

Johnson, M. K. (2020). *Making a Decision on Ethical Decision-Making Models*. All Graduate Theses and Dissertations. 7818. https://digitalcommons.usu.edu/etd/7818

Kim, H., Ji, J., & Kao, D. (2011). Burnout and physical health among social workers: A three-year longitudinal study. *Social Work*, *56*(3), 258–268. https://doi.org/10.1093/sw/56.3.258

Leszcz, M. (2018). The evidence-based group psychotherapist. *Psychoanalytic Inquiry*, *38*, 285–298. https://doi.org/10.1080/07351690.2018.1444853

Leszcz, M., & Kobos, J. C. (2008). Evidence-based group psychotherapy: Using AGPA's practice guidelines to enhance clinical effectiveness. *Journal of Clinical Psychology*, *64*, 1238–1260. https://doi.org/10.1002/jclp.20531

Litam, S. D. A. (2020). "Take your Kung-Flu back to Wuhan": Counseling Asians, Asian Americans, and pacific islanders with race-based trauma related to COVID-19. *The Professional Counselor*, *10*(2), 144–156. https://doi.org/10.15241/sdal.10.2.144

Mills, C. (2014). *Decolonizing global mental health: The psychiatrization of the majority world*. Hove: Routledge.

Morse, G., Salyers, M. P., Rollins, A. L., Monroe-DeVita, M., & Pfahler, C. (2012). Burnout in mental health services: a review of the problem and its remediation. *Administration and Policy in Mental Health, 39*(5), 341–352. https://doi.org/10.1007/s10488-011-0352-1

National Association of Social Workers. (2021). NASW Code of Ethics. https://www.socialworkers.org/About/Ethics/Code-of-Ethics/Code-of-Ethics-English

Ruch, D. A., Heck, K. M., Sheftall, A. H., Fontanella, C. A., Stevens, J., Zhu, M., Horowitz, L. M., Campo, J. V., & Bridge, J. A. (2021). Characteristics and precipitating circumstances of suicide among children aged 5 to 11 years in the United States, 2013–2017. *JAMA Network Open, 4*(7), e2115683. https://doi.org/10.1001/jamanetworkopen.2021.15683

Shechtman, Z. (2006). *Group counseling and psychotherapy with children and adolescents: Theory, research, and practice*. Mahwah, NJ: Lawrence Erlbaum Associates: Mahwah.

Sheppard, T. L. (2017). Evaluation and practice-based evidence. In C. Haen, & S. Aronson (Eds.), *Handbook of child and adolescent group therapy: A practitioner's reference* (pp. 40–49). New York: Routledge.

Somoray, K., Shakespeare-Finch, J., & Armstrong, D. (2017). The impact of personality and workplace belongingness on mental health workers' professional quality of life. *Australian Psychologist, 52*, 52–61.

Sori, C. F., & Hecker, L. L. (2015). Ethical and legal considerations when counselling children and families. *Australian & New Zealand Journal of Family Therapy, 36*(4), 450–464. https://doi.org/10.1002/anzf.1126

Türk, D. (2019). Combined and parallel individual and group therapy—still a red rag? *Group Analysis, 52*(3), 313–329. https://doi.org/10.1177/0533316419849503

Viehl, C., Dispenza, F., McCullough, R., & Guvensel, K. (2017). Burnout among sexual minority mental health practitioners: Investigating correlates and predictors. *Psychology of Sexual Orientation and Gender Diversity, 4*, 354–361.

Walling, M. A. (2021). Suicide contagion. *Current Trauma Reports, 7*(4), 103–114. https://doi.org/10.1007/s40719-021-00219-9

Wendt, D. C., Gone, J. P., & Nagata, D. K. (2015). Potentially harmful therapy and multicultural counseling: Bridging two disciplinary discourses. *The Counseling Psychologist, 43*(3), 334–358. https://doi.org/10.1177/0011000014548280

8 Practical Matters in Child Group Therapy

Tony L. Sheppard

Introduction

Just as therapy groups require grounding in theory, practical issues are also critical to the success of the group. Therapists must consider the who, what, when and where of the group. Groups with children can succeed or fail based upon the therapist's attention to details. Keeping children's therapy groups running requires resourcefulness, creativity and a great deal of energy. The good news is that this can be accomplished with the right mix of resources, awareness of setting-specific challenges and consistent decisions about the content of the group.

Different settings in which groups are conducted require different approaches. A number of settings will be discussed with regard to issues that are unique to that particular way of conducting groups. Further, particularly in working with children, it is critical to think and work systemically. The family system must be taken into account and engaged in order for lasting changes to occur. The child group therapist will be challenged to consider how to carry the improvements noted in the group room outside into the client's natural environment. This is often thought of in terms of the generalizability of growth and change across settings in which the child lives.

As discussed in Chapter 1 of this book, there are a number of presenting issues for which group therapy works very well. A sampling of these presenting issues will be reviewed with ideas for group interventions for each. Additionally, it is important to engage as many of the learning styles as possible for children to get the most benefit from group sessions. The ideas presented in this chapter will be viewed through the lens of engaging multiple intelligences and learning styles. This will provide the child group therapist with ideas that can be adapted to their specific group settings, populations and diversity of cultures.

It is important to consider ownership of the group. Children need to feel that they have a say in what happens in their group. Rule and norm setting in groups is critical to their success and to the safety of their members. Relatedly, it is of the utmost importance to consider the establishment of goals for treatment. This has to be considered both on an individual level and on a group-as-a-whole level. Creative ways of getting children to invest and develop ownership of the group will be discussed. Further, consideration will be given to ways of getting children to identify goals for treatment. A structured approach is required for this since most children don't readily identify appropriate goals for their treatment.

In sum, the goal of this chapter is to catch some of the detail-oriented considerations not readily captured in other chapters. These are:

- **Setting-Specific Issues** (pros and cons of common child group settings, relevant factors for each)

DOI: 10.4324/9781003189701-8

- **Thinking Systemically** (communication with caregivers, generalizing into the child's natural environment)
- **Clinical Presentation-Specific Issues** (samples for unique clinical populations)
- **Logistical Considerations in Child Groups** (goal setting, food)

Setting-Specific Issues

Different settings present different challenges and opportunities. The group therapist must consider the type of setting in which their groups take place. There are unique issues that will impact the way the group is conceptualized, executed and even ended in various settings.

Inpatient Groups

As with any setting, groups in inpatient facilities have both advantages and disadvantages. A primary advantage of inpatient groups is that attendance is often ensured since members are already in the facility. Further, **groups can focus on very specific skills and abilities combining psychoeducation with in-vivo practice in a controlled environment**. Children can use the therapeutic milieu of an inpatient unit to make significant gains. Groups involving family members can often facilitate significant changes on a family systems level in addition to the change that can occur on an individual level.

However, groups in inpatient settings also carry a number of disadvantages. Among these are that children in an acute state often struggle to focus on group therapy. Overworked hospital staff may view group therapy as a burden and not put forth much effort. If there isn't administrative guidance, group therapy might not be integrated into the overall milieu of therapy, thereby limiting its power. The open nature of inpatient groups makes it difficult to achieve the working stage in the group. This refers to the fact that there is a constant rotation of children in and out of the group as patients are admitted and discharged. Finally, as inpatient stays for children become shorter, inpatient groups likely lose even more of their power, changing the focus to predominantly skills-building exercises and psychoeducation. There is likely time to introduce skills and cognitive information, but little time and space to practice and integrate this into a child's repertoire of skills.

Therapy groups in inpatient settings are often characterized by the following:

- Each group session is viewed as a stand-alone meeting, as some members may be discharged or unable to attend subsequent sessions
- Group sessions are typically short, ranging from 15 to 45 minutes (MacLennan in Riester & Kraft, 1986)
- Group sessions are integrated into the overall treatment milieu (MacLennan in Riester & Kraft, 1986)
- Some of the sessions may involve family members in a multifamily format

Groups in Residential Settings

Creeden and Haen (in Haen & Aronson, 2017) note that group therapy has long been a hallmark of residential treatment settings. They also note that groups in these settings often function as subgroups of the numerous groups that exist within residential settings (e.g. academic groups, milieu, program groups, etc.). The authors suggest child group therapists working in this setting must bear in mind a number of key considerations unique to residential systems.

First of all, they note the prevalence of trauma and loss among those in residential facilities. The residential group therapist should have a keen eye toward the existence of these issues. Similar to inpatient settings, it is important in residential settings to ensure integration of the group content into the overall treatment milieu. Creeden and Haen caution against a divide that can exist between milieu staff and therapeutic staff.

Advantages to groups in residential settings include the fact that group members are typically present for all group sessions since they are living in the facility. Further, residential treatment settings allow for more depth-oriented work with clients. The duration of their stay in a given program can permit children to work through issues that they might not be able to address in a shorter-term treatment modality (e.g. inpatient or Intensive Outpatient groups). Finally, there are good opportunities for practice of skills taught and developed in the group setting in the broader milieu of treatment.

The fact that therapy groups within residential settings are often subgroups of other groups as noted above can be a challenge. This can be seen as a disadvantage to these types of groups. Children in residential settings are often together much of the time in the treatment milieu. Therefore, issues that present in the milieu often present in the group sessions and vice versa. There is less separation and delineation between the group boundaries and the rest of the milieu. This can be an asset in that group therapy time can be a time when issues are worked through therapeutically. Conversely, it can present as a liability in that content from the group sessions can spill over into other aspects of the treatment program. It is critical that these issues are addressed not just in the context of the group, but in the overall program. Finally, groups in residential settings can be challenging simply as a function of the acuity of issues faced by children in residential settings.

Groups in the School Setting

Therapy groups in the school setting have many advantages and disadvantages. **A primary advantage of school-based therapy groups is that of convenience and access: Students are already in school and can easily be involved in a group**. Diamond, Gans & Mortola (in Haen & Aronson, 2017) note as well that addressing mental health concerns in school doesn't require parents to provide transportation, which can be a hardship for some families. Further, these authors note that school-based groups afford "access to those children in families who view mental health services as threatening" (p. 206). Additionally, providing school-based groups can help with generalization of skills since children are in the setting where problems may manifest and can readily practice skills both in and out of the group.

Just as there are advantages to school-based groups, disadvantages also exist. Diamond, Gans & Mortola note that primary among these is **time constraints: Scheduling group therapy around academic priorities can be challenging**. Further, there is the issue of stigma, as children may be uncomfortable attending therapy groups in the school setting. Children in school groups have differing levels of dual relationships and may be in groups with close friends, enemies, or "frenemies." **Dual relationships alter group dynamics in school settings and must be attended to throughout the life of school groups**.

There are a number of considerations for the child group therapist conducting school-based therapy groups. Diamond, Gans & Mortola (In Haen & Aronson, 2017) note three primary considerations. First among these is communicating with school personnel. Secondly, they note the importance of understanding and following school policies and procedures. Finally, they state the importance of considering accountability and measurement of goals and progress.

The therapist must work collaboratively with teachers, administrators and parents. It is essential to the success of these groups to have the support of school personnel and parents. The child group therapist must be sensitive to the fact that some therapeutic work and interventions may not be appropriate for the school setting. Following a group session, children must be able to return to class and engage in academic work. Therapeutic work that evokes significant emotion may interfere with their ability to do so. Stark et al., writing in Stoiber and Kratochwill (1998), discuss a school-based group for depressed children which has a strictly cognitive focus due to concerns about the stimulation of too much emotion in the school setting.

Time frames of group sessions in schools may differ from those in other settings. Due to the need to work around the child's academic priorities, sessions may vary in length from the traditional 60- or 90-minute formats. Stark et al. (in Stoiber & Kratochwill, 1998) report conducting sessions as short as 30 minutes with younger children. Confidentiality presents a challenge in school settings. It is often extremely difficult to maintain complete confidentiality in school settings. The logistics of taking children from the classroom to the group space will sometimes make it obvious that the child attends a therapy group. Attention should be paid to minimizing the impact of this.

Therapists should be particularly sensitive to any stigma attached to group involvement.

MacLennan, writing in Riester and Kraft (1986), notes, "The reputation the group therapy program develops in the school will be critical for the success of the groups" (p. 92). Therapists based in schools must work to reduce the stigma attached to psychotherapy.

Groups in Community Agencies

Gillespie and Iklas (writing in Stoiber & Kratochwill, 1998) discuss groups for children and adolescents in the community context. These authors define community agencies as:

- Community mental health centers
- Hospitals providing outpatient services
- Schools
- Head Start agencies
- Other community agencies

Such settings offer a number of advantages and disadvantages. Advantages of groups in a community agency setting include accessibility to many people due to the community-based nature of these groups. Often there is funding that permits a number of groups to run at any given time (e.g. Medicaid, Commercial Insurance, grants, etc.). Available funding also increases accessibility for children who may otherwise not have access to mental health groups. Further, **these groups can be quite responsive to the needs of the community in that they can deal with topics and problems frequently seen in these settings** (e.g. anger focused groups, groups for children with ADHD, Parent Child Interaction Therapy groups, etc.). Larger agencies are able to create new groups with existing clients to address identified needs.

As with all settings, there are also disadvantages of groups in community agencies. Gillespie and Iklas (writing in Stoiber & Kratochwill, 1998) state, "In the reality of implementation, community mental health center (CMHC) practice has fallen short of (these) ideals" (p. 33). These agencies often do not offer services that meet the needs of their communities. These authors note that most CMHC services focus on existing pathology and do little to take a preventative approach. Community agencies may also encounter client- or setting-specific difficulties with families and clinicians who are attempting to balance multiple responsibilities or challenges. As a result, attendance, follow-through with interventions outside of groups and busy therapist schedules remain practical challenges for groups in community settings.

Groups in Private Practice

Group psychotherapy with children can work very well in a private practice setting. Advantages of groups in a private practice setting include the lack of stigma often associated with agencies. Children and their families might feel comfortable attending a group in a private practice setting whereas an agency setting might carry more stigma. Some agencies have a more institutional feel and might carry stigma as a result. Further, the therapist is often free from the funding, paperwork, and administrative constraints present in agencies. Groups in private practice can offer clinicians an increase in income, particularly where reimbursement rates are fair. Finally, this setting may offer more opportunities for doing preventive work with children and their families.

Private practice groups are not without their disadvantages. There can be funding issues in the private practice setting as well. Insurance reimbursement for group therapy is often minimal. Depending upon reimbursement rates, groups may not be as financially profitable for the therapist as seeing children individually. In those settings where insurance is not accepted for payment, some families cannot afford to pay for group therapy on an ongoing basis. Other challenges noted by MacLennan (1986, writing in Riester & Kraft) include the challenge of getting enough referrals to an outpatient, private practice to fill a group or groups. There can be space constraints in private practice settings since a large room is required for groups. While some community agencies might provide transportation and children are already present in school settings, those attending groups in private practice might experience difficulties with transportation.

Strategies for success with children's groups in private practice are important to consider. Pojman, writing in Haen and Aronson (2017), notes the importance of communication with parents and guardians in the private practice setting. He recommends brief phone calls, periodic or regular newsletters to parents or parent meetings (p. 225). Technology also permits the use of e-mail communication with parents.

Short-term, time-limited groups (6–12 week sessions) often work well in private practice. From a marketing perspective, therapists often find that topical groups are easier to promote. This would include groups such as Anger Management, Social Skills, Divorce Groups, Grief Groups, etc. It is of significant importance in the private practice setting to effectively market groups to potential referral sources. These might include teachers and other school officials, pediatricians and other mental health professionals such as outpatient therapists, inpatient facilities and psychiatrists.

An important part of a marketing strategy for group therapists in private practice is setting oneself apart as an expert group therapist. Becoming a local expert in group therapy involves consistent time and investment with other professionals in the area. This is frequently time invested in one's work, however, since the payoff can be great. The following activities can help promote the practitioner as an expert in group psychotherapy:

- Present on group topics at professional meetings
- Become a Certified Group Psychotherapist (CGP) or obtain advanced training in group work with children
- Write an article about groups in a local trade newsletter or other resource

Working Systemically

Group therapy with children requires a layer of attention that is often not required in adult group work. Children can neither consent to nor involve themselves in a therapy group of their own accord. The child group therapist must consider the role that caregivers play in the child's treatment and in the overall approach to the group. Caregivers can include myriad people in the child's life, but when we refer to caregivers, we are typically referencing that child's legal guardian or guardians. **To work systemically is to consider – and at times intervene with – the broader environments in which children exist every day**. As opposed to adult groups which would rarely contact people in a client's life, child group clinicians may be in contact with caregivers, school teachers, school counselors, grandparents, camp counselors and others.

First and foremost, group leaders must secure the consent of a child's legal guardian in order to engage the child in treatment. Therapists should be aware of the laws regarding this in the jurisdiction in which they practice. Family therapy theorists have long advocated a systemic approach to therapy (Haley, 1991; Kerr & Bowen, 1988; Minuchin & Fishman, 1981). This is particularly important to working with children. Children are often reliant upon their parents or other caregivers to bring them to group sessions. Regular attendance in a group is ensured when parents and other adults are invested in the group and its goals. Corey et al. (2015) note that it is important to keep parents and other caregivers informed of what is happening in the group in order to avoid misperceptions about the group, its goals, and its purposes (p. 51). Making parents and other adults aware of the work children are doing in group has a number of advantages:

* They can support children in their work toward goals.
* There is a higher likelihood that skills learned in a group will generalize if adults in other settings (home, school, etc.) can reinforce the use of these.
* Parents and other adults can offer the group therapist valuable feedback on the progress of the child.

Beyond keeping caregivers aware of what is happening in the group once it is meeting, there is the issue of helping them to understand the purposes of the group prior to its start. This is an important part of framing the goals of the group so that caregivers know what to expect from their child's involvement. Tollison and Synatschk (2007) suggest the following methods for educating parents and other collateral adults about the child's therapy group (p. 43):

* Announcements at faculty and PTA meetings
* Newsletters
* Flyers and information brochures
* Websites

Getting caregiver buy-in to the group is a complicated endeavor. It is important to address this in an initial meeting with the caregivers. Orientation to the overarching goals of the group is a key part of this process. One way of accomplishing this is through both verbal and written means.

In a private practice located in a metropolitan area the group therapists have identified three broad areas that are addressed in their groups. These include (1) Self-control-Becoming aware of one's own emotions and learning to regulate them; (2) Interpersonal Skills-Learning

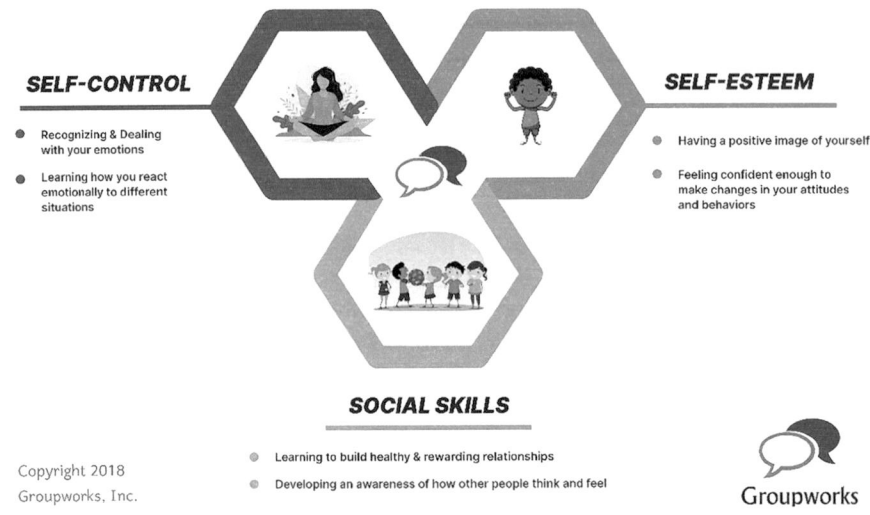

Group Therapy at Groupworks addresses three very
important areas in the lives of children and teens!

Regardless of the problems faced by youth, improvement in
these three core areas helps build a healthy life and future.

SELF-CONTROL
- Recognizing & Dealing with your emotions
- Learning how you react emotionally to different situations

SELF-ESTEEM
- Having a positive image of yourself
- Feeling confident enough to make changes in your attitudes and behaviors

SOCIAL SKILLS
- Learning to build healthy & rewarding relationships
- Developing an awareness of how other people think and feel

Copyright 2018
Groupworks, Inc.

Groupworks

Figure 8.1 Marketing Example

to form healthy relationships with others and (3) Positive Self-Esteem-Developing a positive sense of what one has to offer. These core goals are communicated across various platforms with parents including the following:

- The practice website
- In printed materials provided to parents in the initial intake
- Verbally communicated at the beginning of the initial intake

Communicating these core goals in this way ensures that parents understand the goals of the group. The following graphic assists in communicating these core group goals as well (Figure 8.1):

Effective groups offer some structured mechanism for ensuring communication between the group leader and significant adults in the child's life. This involves both communication about what happens in the group sessions and information about the goals and purposes of the group. Didactic information provided to caregivers might include educational materials focused on a specific problem or issue, summaries of issues relevant to group sessions and general educational materials for parents on generalizing gains and applying skills from the group.

Communication with caregivers regarding goals and progress toward them is of critical importance. Just as the group leader works with children to determine the content and goals of each session, the leader should elicit input from caregivers on issues facing the child. Use of goal sheets, rating forms, feedback forms and informal notes can help to keep information flowing both to and from caregivers. The use of caregiver-feedback sessions periodically can be of benefit as well. This would involve a brief meeting with parents or guardians to discuss progress toward goals and to set new goals once others are met.

Finally, there might be a need to share information about the group with others in the child's life beyond caregivers. This might include teachers, school counselors, individual therapists and others involved with the child's treatment. Some of the ideas presented in this chapter, particularly in the subsequent section, can be used for this purpose in addition to being shared with caregivers.

Parent Feedback Sessions

The Kids Club group program is an open-ended group for children. This program involves Parent Feedback Sessions that occur every 8 weeks during a child's involvement in the program. This facilitates the two-way communication described above. The group leader/s communicate the following to the caregiver/s in these sessions:

* Progress Seen
* Current Goals
* Significant Concerns about the Child
* Recommendations about the child's involvement in the program (e.g. whether or not they continue their involvement for another eight weeks)

The group leader/s elicit the following information from the caregiver/s:

* Caregiver impressions of progress
* Changes in medications and other treatments
* Parent Goals for the Child
* Updates on the following
  ◦ School Functioning
  ◦ Family Functioning
  ◦ Friends/Social Functioning
  ◦ Engagement with Hobbies/Interests
* Caregiver Impressions about the child's involvement in the program

Sample Communications with Parents and Caregivers

The following are examples of weekly communications that are sent to caregivers of children involved in groups in a private practice setting. The intent is to keep parents apprised of what is being addressed in the group and to provide them with ideas on continuing this work at home. Not only does this help with caregiver investment in the group, it also assists with the generalization of new skills and growth outside the group. When caregivers are able to prompt children to practice new skills in various settings (e.g. at home, on the playground, in sports, etc.), these skills begin to generalize outside the group room with greater efficiency. Caregivers also benefit from hearing about the work that is going on in the group setting. This facilitates their knowing that problem areas and areas of deficit are being addressed by the group leader. It should be noted that only general information is shared in these communications. Specific information about individuals is never shared in this format due to confidentiality concerns.

Eye Contact & Body Language

We'll be working on eye contact, body language and focusing attention during this session. The group will discuss the importance of eye contact when you're talking with someone. We'll also discuss why it can sometimes be hard and scary to do this. Along with this, we will consider the fact that we communicate more with our bodies than we do with words. The kids will have several opportunities to practice each of these skills.

We'll use visual aids and a program called *Clue Cards* to help us practice these skills. This practice will build up to next week when we'll challenge the children to have a group conversation on a chosen topic.

How Can You Help At Home….

• In group, we use non-verbal cues like cupping a hand behind the ear, pointing toward a speaker, etc. to help the kids remember where their attention should be. We also use visual cues such as the 'spotlight.'
• Focus on body language, eye contact, and tone of voice with your child this week. Remember…coach, don't nag or criticize!
• One of the most important skills that we try to develop with the kids is that of *Ignoring*! We challenge them to ignore (or filter out) distractions. Simply reminding them to ignore annoying distractions can be a powerful intervention.
• Offer rewards for practice of these skills in different situations and settings. (Small ones…)

Anger

Anger is a difficult emotion that everyone feels. Kids often struggle with managing this emotion in a healthy way. Today's group session will teach kids some important skills for managing anger. The emphasis is on managing the emotion, not getting rid of it.

We will discuss some of our anger triggers as well as the ways that we express anger. Group members will be encouraged to think in terms of 'clean' and 'dirty' anger. The latter refers to healthy expressions and the former refers to not-so-healthy expressions.

We will create a handout as a group with ideas for expressing anger in 'clean' ways. We'll make copies and send them home, so make sure you take a look!

To Continue the Work At Home

• Help your child practice these skills when the steam is building.
• Add to the list as a family when you discover new ways of expressing 'clean' anger.

These specific examples on the topics of Eye Contact & Body Language and Anger offer parents a window into the group in which their child is involved. The advice on how to continue to work at home is seen as increasing parent investment in their child's treatment.

Objectives and Sample Activities for Various Types of Groups

While it is beyond the scope of this chapter to offer an exhaustive list of activities for different presenting issues, it is helpful to see how common presenting issues might be worked with during group sessions. There is a rich array of books that offer issue-specific activities that are amenable to children's groups. In the section below, common presenting problems are provided along with objectives and sample activities for each. Attention is paid to engaging different learning styles and sensory modalities. Case examples are used to highlight specific activities.

Anger and Impulse Control

Objectives for the group

- Improve frustration tolerance
- Teach the use of I-statements
- Improve self-esteem
- Teach children to stop and think before acting
- Improve peer relations

Sample Activity

- Teach children to use an anger thermometer model of thinking about and working with anger
- Have them act out the different levels of anger
- Use role play to teach appropriate management of anger and "moving down" the anger thermometer

Case Example

A group that is working on anger is engaged in some psychoeducation about anger and how it affects members. Using an Anger Thermometer poster in the group room, children are engaged in acting out each level of anger paying attention to how they feel and how it manifests for them. The instruction goes as follows:

Group Leader: "I want everyone to imagine that someone in your class at school or maybe your sibling at home if you have one does something that really annoys you. In fact, you move up to the "Annoyed" level on the Anger Thermometer. Now, I'd like for you to each take a turn to tell us how this feels for you. Where do you feel it in your body?"

<Each member takes a turn to say how they feel this level of anger in their body. They can also be encouraged to share a thought that they're having as well>

Now, using slow motion, I'd like for each of you to take a turn to show us how you would look when you're annoyed. Remember, this is a low level of anger, so don't show us your full anger yet.

<Each member gets a turn to demonstrate how they would look at the Annoyed level on the Anger Thermometer. Children are asked to use slow motion so that there aren't sudden movements that could be scary or threatening. Group members are asked to act out each of the levels of the Anger Thermometer in turn until all have been addressed. The group leader comments on similarities and differences in anger expression among group members, taking care not to judge a members' anger expression>

Note: The phrase "I Flipped My Lid!" is based upon the work of Daniel Siegel and his "Handy Model of the Brain" (Siegel, 2013, pp. 102, 103; Siegel, 2020, pp. 36, 37) (Figure 8.2).

Attention Deficit Hyperactivity Disorder

Objectives for the group

- Improve frustration tolerance
- Improve self-esteem
- Teach children to stop and think before acting
- Teach techniques for managing attention and focus
- Improve peer relations

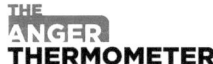

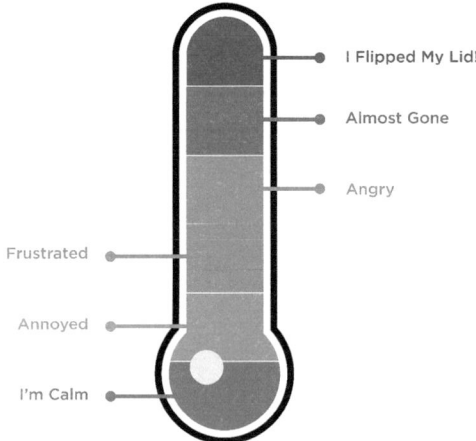

Figure 8.2 Anger Thermometer

Sample Activity

- Place items on a table and give children instructions on what to do with the items
- Gradually increase the instructions from one to three consecutive
- E.g. First round – Place the toy bear on the paper; Second round – Place the toy snake on the paper and pick up the blue cup; Third round – Place the pencil on the floor, turn the blue cup upside down and pick up the toy snake
- Give group members a prize for being "a good listener"!

Case Example

A children's group is engaged in a bowling game using soft bowling pins and a plastic bowling ball. This activity usually spans several sessions that culminate in a group game of bowling where children are divided up into teams. The initial stage of this game involves learning to bowl. In this stage, children are encouraged to practice bowling and are given coaching by both the group leaders and by peers. In order to develop focusing and attending skills, group members have to wait when it is their turn to bowl until the leader holds up a sign that reads "Go!" This encourages pausing and taking one's time prior to rolling the ball. The purpose of practice rounds is stated as learning to be a better bowler, but also to be better at practicing "good sportspersonship."

What follows is a parent communication that was sent during the bowling emphasis in the group:

BEING A GOOD SPORT

This week in Kids Club we reviewed what it means to be a good sport and get along with others.

For the activity this week, the members participated in a bowling game. Bowling in group offers members the opportunity to practice healthy competition, let go when we make a mistake, cheer each other on with positive words and encourage ourselves in a positive way. During the game, there was some level of frustration due to not hitting the bowling pins, and the kids were encouraged to offer each other advice in a kind and supportive way. By practicing healthy competition, kids will be able to take these skills and apply them to other games, sports and situations at home and at school! We also continue to work on some of the basics of social and friendship skills. It feels good to help this group develop these skills that will help them navigate the world better!

In order to carry on these lessons at home, play games with your children that have a clear winner. Sometimes by playing games, kids do not think they are actually learning anything but in fact they are! While playing a game, encourage your child to think positively, to cheer on their opponent, to compete in a healthy way and to practice positivity if they lose. Learning to lose well is such an important life lesson!

Depression and Anxiety

Objectives for the group

- Develop better awareness of feelings
- Teach children a feelings language
- Teach positive thinking patterns
- Develop healthy communication patterns
- Improve self-esteem
- Improve peer relations

Sample Activity

- Engage children in making a list of "how to make my bad days better"
- Have each child choose one way that they will practice for the week
- Follow up on how this activity worked for them

Case Example

The group leaders set up a laptop, tablet or computer in the group room. Members of the group are encouraged to brainstorm ways of "making my bad days better." Group members take turns typing their ideas into the computer. They are guided to add clip-art to the project and a "handout" is created. These are printed and members are encouraged to circle the ideas that they want to practice during the upcoming week.

Interpersonal Skills

Objectives for the group

- Develop better awareness of feelings
- Teach children a feelings language
- Improve self-esteem
- Improve peer relations
- Increase children's social microskills to better connect with peers
- Improve emotional regulation during social connection

Sample Group Activity

- Provide children with an interview form (simple)
- Allow them to interview another group member
- Have members introduce the member to the group using their interview form

Groups for Children Diagnosed with Autism Spectrum Disorder (ASD)

Objectives for the group

- Build a sense of universality among the children with regard to their experiences
- Develop better awareness of feelings
- Teach children a feelings language
- Improve self-esteem
- Improve peer relations

Sample Activity

- Play emotions charades where children are encouraged to act out emotions
- When children struggle with this, engage the group in problem solving to assist with emotional awareness

Children Who Have Experienced Trauma and/or Abuse

Objectives for the group

- Build a sense of universality among the children with regard to their experiences
- Develop better awareness of feelings and a sense of personal security
- Teach children a feelings language
- Improve self-esteem
- Improve peer relations

Sample Activity

- Use creative arts such as painting or drawing to assist with emotional expression

Clinical Example

Group members are given colored pencils and pastels and are encouraged to draw their "safe place." This is a space where they feel safe from their trauma and their fears. Members then get a chance to share their drawings with each other.

Parenting Groups and Multifamily Groups

Objectives for the group

- Teach parenting skills
- Increase self-efficacy of parents
- Develop a sense of universality with regard to parental struggles

Sample Activity

•   Have families join together in playing a game

Clinical Example

A small group of three children and their caregivers are engaged in playing a game such as charades or Apples to Apples, Jr. When children struggle with rules, boundaries or self-expression, the game is paused and all members are engaged in problem solving in order to assist the child who is struggling.

Ownership, Investment, Rules

Helping children to engage with group therapy involves giving them some autonomy in certain aspects of their group experience. A number of authors suggest that involving children in decision-making about the group builds ownership and motivation (Corey et al., 2018; Shechtman, 2007; Smead, 1995; Tollison & Synatschk, 2007). This building of motivation helps to establish group cohesion, which is essential in healthy, working groups. Such involvement can include:

•   Allowing children to assist in establishing group rules
•   Having children participate in the naming of the group
•   Allowing members to select activities
•   Getting input from members about the types of refreshments offered (Mishna et al., 2002)
•   Encouraging members to set both group and individual goals

Rules of the group will likely change depending on the setting. For example, more rules might be necessary in inpatient and residential settings due to the acuity of the issues faced by the children. Likewise, fewer rules might be needed in an outpatient setting such as a private practice, school or agency setting.

Sample ground rules for an outpatient children's group might include the following:

•   Use words not actions
•   Listen and pay attention
•   Keep hands and feet to yourself
•   Support others

Case Example

The Kids Club group, a group that focuses on improving members' self-awareness, self-esteem and social skills uses the following group rules that are posted in the group room:

1   Use nice words & actions to show respect for others
2   Follow directions
3   It's OK to feel!
4   Use your listening eyes, ears, mouth & body
5   Help each other feel good
6   Be flexible
7   Keep our bodies to ourselves

Table 8.1 Sample Children's Group Activities

Examples of Structured Activities in Children's Groups
Creative Arts Interventions
Role Plays
Games
Worksheets
Brainstorming Sessions
Multimedia Activities
Physical Activities
Practice of Skills

The Use of Structured Activities

Children's groups are more likely than adolescent and adult groups to rely on structured activities. As discussed in previous chapters of this book, children need to move, play, dance and create in order to learn. It is the true definition of learning by doing. As noted previously, these structured activities don't have to take away from a process focus in children's groups. The process often emerges from the interaction in the activity. The table below presents just some of the possible structured activities that can be employed in groups with children (Table 8.1).

Creative Arts Interventions

Creative arts interventions allow for the engagement of multiple intelligences and learning modalities. They also engage children in both play and creativity; two engagement and learning modes that are primary in their experience of the world. Dean & Landis (in Haen & Aronson, 2017) note that creative arts interventions allow the expression of a range of emotions and that they can help with cutting through resistances. Most children enjoy the arts and it can be a way for them to relate and learn outside the typical channels of strictly cognition and dialogue.

Examples of creative arts interventions include:

- Role Play
- Visual art
  - Drawing
  - Painting
  - Coloring
  - Making art items
- Movement
  - Dance
  - Play
  - Sociometry
  - Games

Role play is a broad term used to describe a variety of different activities and interventions. Corey et al. (2018) note that role playing by group members allows them to "learn how to express themselves more effectively, test reality, and practice new behavior" (p. 333). Children enjoy taking on personas and acting things out. Further, Carnabucci (2014) points out that "the brain does not distinguish between experiences of daily life and experiences that are structured within the psychodrama treatment room, classroom or other protected setting" (p. 24). In other words, acting out situations allows the brain to process them in similar ways to how it processes real-life situations. Invaluable learning can occur from role-playing situations.

Movement, such as that involved in role play, is essential for children's learning and growth. With regard to play specifically, for example, Carnabucci (2014) notes that it literally changes the brain in so many helpful ways. Movement can take a number of forms in children's groups. The following is an example of a role play activity that can be used in a group.

Children involved in an 8-week group for anger management are encouraged to act out scenarios related to the expression of anger. The tone set in the group is one of playfulness in taking on new roles and practicing behaviors learned in the group. A stage area is identified for the children so that the activity has a sense of awe and showpersonship. Members are given scenarios that involve anger and are engaged in creating responses to them. They are encouraged to act them out using both 'dirty' and 'clean' anger. The former involves acting the scenario out in a way that expresses anger in an unhealthy manner. The latter involves acting out the scenario in a manner that expresses anger in a healthy way. A note with regard to the former is that children are sometimes asked to act out certain aspects of the situation in slow motion or silently. This guards against unhealthy anger being expressed in a threatening manner. It also helps in avoiding triggering any trauma or sensitivity symptoms on other group members.

Visual art interventions allow for children to engage in learning and growth using art as a way of communicating. Art interventions break down barriers among group members and between the group members and the group leaders. Dean & Landis (in Haen & Aronson, 2017) note that "artwork becomes an entry point through which therapist and client can begin a verbal dialogue" (p. 126). In a group setting, this dialogue opens up among group members as well. Most children feel at ease when drawing, coloring, painting or creating crafts and art projects. As stated previously in this book, the group process unfolds through this expression. The following is an example of an art project being used in a group setting:

Children involved in an ongoing process group focused on depression and anxiety are engaged in an art project that involves making a coping box. The creation of these boxes spans several sessions with a different component as a focus during each given session.

First, children are encouraged to draw a picture of something that helps them calm down. This can be a person, place, pet, etc. They are provided with pencils, colored pencils, markers and crayons for this part of the activity. Group process unfolds around the sharing of the materials and how the children respond to the activity. Group leaders facilitate this group process. For example, if two members want the same marker, this is negotiated. Further, if a member becomes upset because they "messed up" their drawing, the leader facilitates processing this and utilizing some of the coping strategies taught in the group.

Second, members are encouraged to write a list of their favorite coping skills and to decorate that list using pictures from magazines, stickers and scrapbooking supplies.

Finally, members are provided with art supplies and encouraged to decorate the actual box in which their coping items will be stored.

Other ideas for these boxes include making calming jars out of glitter, glue and water, making slime and placing it in a jar.

Since children *learn by doing*, games are a very important part of children's groups. While there are games that are therapeutically oriented, there is also great value in playing games that are not inherently therapeutic. Some of the classic therapeutically oriented games are *The Ungame: Kids Version* and *The Talking Feeling Doing Game*. While these can be valuable resources for children's groups, group members often respond just as well or even better to games that are not inherently therapeutic. It is important for the group therapist to keep in mind that any game can be therapeutic if it permits the acquisition or practice of new skills. Games such as these that are frequently used in children's groups include the following:

- Apples to Apples, Junior
- Whonu by Cranium
- Uno
- Jenga
- Exploding Kittens
- Superfight
- Pictionary, Junior

Technology offers another common route child clinicians can use to effectively engage with child groups. Example games using technology include (and are certainly not limited to) the following:

- Among Us
- Mario Kart
- Minecraft
- Roblox
- Just Dance

The child group therapist is cautioned that for these games to be therapeutic there have to be goals associated with them. The group leader needs an appropriate rationale for playing a specific game in a specific session. For example, child group members could work as a team or in dyads to co-create a design within Minecraft. Thus, a video game could be used to work on social skills in a fun, collaborative task. The rationale for a particular game is often associated with the acquisition or practice of specific skills. Mario Kart could be used to practice frustration tolerance or social skills when losing a game. Apples to Apples, Junior can be used to practice interpersonal skills by applying knowledge of a group member to the strategy of effectively choosing a card for a specific member. The following clinical examples offer insight into how games such as those above might be employed with an appropriate rationale in a group setting.

Case Example

In the initial stage of a children's therapy group, the group therapist employs the game Whonu as a way of helping the group to get to know each other and to begin to build some group cohesion. This game involves cards with items listed on them. Group members choose cards/items that they think another group member will like. This member then ranks the items on the cards from their least favorite to their favorite. The group leader can begin linking members who like or dislike certain items. For example, if the card says 'Pizza' and someone ranks that one as a favorite, the group leader can say, 'Who else in our group really likes pizza?' Likewise, if the card says 'sushi' and someone ranks that as their least favorite item, the group leader can say, 'Who else in our group really doesn't like sushi?' This can be an initial way of linking group members and helping them find things in common. Further, it can allow members to begin to practice important skills such as frustration tolerance and letting go when their item is not ranked highly by other members of the group.

Case Example

During the working stage of a group, the game Jenga can be used for a number of purposes including building self-confidence and helping members face fears. With regard to the former, each member is encouraged to make a positive self-statement when they pull a block from the tower. Using Jenga to help anxious members face fears involves helping them to face the fear that the tower will fall. Using psychoeducation to help members understand that the tower will fall and that this is OK is the focus of this activity. The group leader helps members to normalize the fear that the tower will fall and to engage with the game anyway.

In each of these examples, the game serves a clear purpose that is consistent with the goals of the group and its members. This exemplifies how games that don't have an inherent therapeutic focus can be meaningfully employed in the work of the group.

Play is central to the lives of children. Therefore, it only makes sense that it would be a key component of their treatment. Groups with children need a playful tone. As discussed in previous chapters, the child group therapist needs a sense of spontaneity and playfulness in order to be successful with children. Whether it is a game or a collection of toys, the child group room must be equipped for play. Just as with any aspect of a child therapy group, the degree of structure of the play involved can vary depending upon the group, its stages of development and the purpose of the play. There have been examples of rather structured play presented in this chapter (e.g. the bowling game). The following clinical example presents a less structured use of play in a group setting with children. It is based upon the model used in Slavson's Activity Group Therapy (Slavson, 1979).

Clinical Example

During the working stage of a group for children, members are engaged in a session that involves free play. Several play areas are set up in the room. These areas include Uno cards, Legos, board games, a Marble shooting game, and an art area. Members are encouraged to divide up into small groups of at least two to play together. At the beginning of the session, key skills that have been taught in the group are reviewed and members are encourage to practice these as they play. These might include (1) Being a good sport, (2) Problem solving, (3) Anger Control and (4) Using Words and Not Actions with each other. The group leaders are available to assist members in practicing these skills when called upon. Group leaders will intervene if problems arise and members don't ask for help.

Goal Setting

Agreeing upon goals for therapy is an essential part of its success. Numerous authors including Corey et al. (2018) and Yalom and Leszcz (2021) stress the importance of the identification of goals in member success in the group. Dumais (in Haen & Aronson, 2017) notes that goal identification is an important part of the group contract with group members and their parents or guardians. He suggests that input from both youth and parents and guardians is necessary since young children might have difficulty identifying appropriate goals for themselves. Further, Dumais suggests reframing goals in youth-friendly terms such as "staying strong" or "becoming a warrior with words" (p. 32).

Smead (1995) delineates two broad categories of goals (pp. 107–112). Leader goals are those goals articulated by the group leader. Member goals are those goals articulated by the child. Both are to be used in determining what is addressed in the therapy. Children will require input from group leaders in setting appropriate goals. Goals for a therapy group exist on two levels: Group-as-a-whole goals and Individual Goals.

- Group-as-a-whole goals
  - Those shared by the entire group
    For example: A group goal for a single session might be to practice cooperation and sharing so that the group can earn a reward.
    For example: A broader group goal might be to work across several sessions to create a 'positive thinking' banner for the group room.
- Individual goals
  - A goal or goals held by an individual member of the group

For example: A child might have a goal of reducing the number of time-outs received at home for shouting.

For example: A child might have a goal of not interrupting or speaking out of turn for an entire group session.

Dumais brings in an important point with regard to goal setting in that children struggle to identify goals for themselves due to their lack of self-awareness. This process needs a greater degree of structure than simply employing a "What is your goal for group" approach. Group leaders might consider using a goals menu or some other way of prompting members to set appropriate goals. Such a tool lists common goals in a given group (in this case an interpersonally focused group that involves children with a number of presenting problems) and children are asked to identify which of these goals they'd like to achieve. The following provides a sample of a Goals Menu and describes how this might be employed in a group setting.

During the first session of a group, the group leaders hand out copies of the group goals menu on clipboards. Members are asked to place a check-mark beside goals that they'd like to "get better at in this group." They are then asked to circle their "top three" goals. These are the things they "want the most and would like to start with." Typically, the group leader would read the goals out loud as members review the handout. Members are then asked to share some of their goals with the group. Group leaders can use this input to begin planning the sessions of the group. This form can be repeated at various intervals throughout the life of the group in order to ensure that goals align with the content of the sessions.

For children, it has been noted that it is important to get input from parents, guardians and other caregivers. This menu could also be given to them either in the waiting room or in an initial visit. This ensures that the goals of the adults in the child's life align with what is being addressed in the group sessions (Figure 8.3).

Food & Snacks

Mishna et al. (2002) and Hariton (in Haen & Aronson, 2017) note that food served in a therapy group helps to set a nurturing tone. While not all group therapists will choose to have food as a component of their therapy groups, it is an important topic to address. Groups that are offered in the community (in private practices, agencies, etc.) often occur immediately after school at a time when children might be hungry. Therefore, offering food can help to meet a need that children might have coming into the group setting.

Grover (in Haen & Aronson, 2017) suggests that members be engaged in the planning of group snacks. This author poses a number of questions for the group to consider when planning to have food as a part of the group:

*   What kind of snack do group members want?
*   At what point in the group should snacks be served?
*   Would group members like to make snacks? (p. 314)

Other important considerations with regard to food include the following:

*   Is the group space conducive to serving food? Is there a kitchen nearby? Are serving utensils available if needed?
*   Is the group leader fully aware of any food allergies? This is of critical importance since food allergies can cause very significant health issues for children.

Group Goals Menu - Kids Club

Name _____   **Date** _____

Make Better Choices

Learn to Sit Still and Pay Attention Better

Think Before I Do & Say Things

Control My Anger

Learn to Make New Friends

Get Along with My Brother/Sister Better

Calm Myself Down When I'm Upset

Feel Better About Myself

Learn to Make my Bad Days Better

Listen to my Parents and Do What they Say

Learn more about My Feelings

Learn to Control my Worries Better

Keep my Hands and Feet to Myself

Talk to the Group about Something that has been Bothering Me

(Write your Own Goal)

Figure 8.3 Group Goals Menu

- Has parental consent been obtained for offering food? It should be noted that some parents control their children's diets for various reasons including food allergies, dietary restrictions, personal preference, religious reasons, etc. It is essential to ensure that these are known and that parents have consented to the offering of snacks and to the specific snack being offered to their child.

- Is the snack consistent with the overall goals of the group? Depending upon the goals of the group, a snack can take up a large portion of the group's time. Is this consistent with the goals of the group?

The following is an example of how a snack can be integrated into a children's group effectively:

A social skills group for children involves a snack each week that consists of cookies and juice boxes. There is a kitchen adjacent to the group room and members take turns assisting the group leaders in preparing, serving and cleaning up after the group snack. As suggested by Hariton (in Haen and Aronson, 2017), the snacktime involves the "news of the week" at which time "children share something about their week" (p. 362). Activities such as this can become very important shared rituals in a group. In this case, it becomes part of the opening or convening ritual of the group. Group process interventions are used to deal with any conflicts or disagreements that arise around the food or the snack. For example, a group could be engaged in group problem solving when they can't agree on what flavor of cookies or juice boxes to serve in the group. Further, members can learn important skills from the serving of the snack to each other.

Exercises

1   Choose a setting for groups such as private practice, residential facility, inpatient facility, etc. Consider the details of beginning a group in that setting.
2   Choose a population or presenting issue (e.g., ADHD, anxiety, etc.) and consider the following with regard to proposing a group focusing on it. Discuss the following in relation to the group:
    1   Length of the sessions
    2   Duration (open-ended versus time-limited)
    3   Structure of the sessions
    4   Physical configuration of the space
    5   Activities and interventions
    6   Working systemically with parents and guardians
    7   Basic rules for the group
3   Consider ways to engage multiple modalities of learning to develop skills for a given presenting issue (e.g. children with ADHD, children on the Autism Spectrum, Anger Management groups, process-oriented groups with children, etc.).

Summary

Practical matters in children's groups matter! While it is not possible to cover every setting or issue that might arise in a therapy group, it is important to think about the more pragmatic side of group therapy with children relevant to the settings in which you practice. Clinicians who are well grounded in theory, but who have not planned for the more practical aspects of therapy, will not be successful in their work in child group therapy. The child group therapist is challenged to view some of these practical decisions as the fun part of therapy. Planning the details of groups such as structured activities, engaging caregivers and setting of goals can be an opportunity to engage the clinician's sense of creativity, spontaneity and passion for the work.

The information contained in this chapter along with the group proposal presented in Chapter 6 challenge the child group therapist to consider important details about the structure of their group. The current chapter serves as a resource for the group therapist who desires to complete a proposal on a group they are considering. Further, even seasoned clinicians are challenged to consider some of these important practical details in running their groups.

References

Carnabucci, K. (2014). *Show and tell psychodrama: Skills for therapists, coaches, teachers, leaders.* Lancaster, PA: Nusanto Publishing.

Corey, G., Callahan, P., & Russell, J. M. (2015). *Group techniques.* Boston, MA: Cengage Learning.

Corey, M. S., Corey, G., & Corey, C. (2018). *Groups: Process and practice.* Boston, MA: Cengage Learning.

Haen, C., & Aronson, S. (2017). *Handbook of child and adolescent group therapy: A practitioner's reference.* New York: Routledge.

Haley, J. (1991). *Problem-solving therapy.* San Francisco, CA: Jossey-Bass.

Kerr, M. E., & Bowen, M. (1988). *Family evaluation: An approach based on Bowen theory.* Tempe, AZ: Norton.

Minuchin, S., & Fishman, H. C. (1981). *Family therapy techniques.* Cambridge, MA: HUP.

Mishna, F., Muskat, B., & Schamess, G. (2002). *Food for thought: The use of food in group therapy with children and adolescents. International Journal of Group Psychotherapy, 52*(1), 27–47.

Riester, A. E., & Kraft, I. A. (1986). *Child group psychotherapy: Future tense.* Madison, CT: International Universities Press.

Shechtman, Z. (2007). *Group counseling and psychotherapy with children and adolescents: Theory, research, and Practice.* New York: Routledge.

Siegel, D. J. (2013). *Brainstorm. The power and purpose of the teenage brain.* London: Jeremy P. Tarcher/Penguin.

Siegel, D. J. (2020). *The developing mind: How relationships and the brain interact to shape who we are.* New York: Guilford Press.

Slavson, S. R. (1979). *Dynamics of group psychotherapy*: Ed. in consultation with the author by Mortimer Schiffer. Aronson.

Stoiber, K. C., & Kratochwill, T. R. (1998). *Handbook of group intervention for children and families.* Boston, MA: Allyn and Bacon.

Tollison, P. K., Synatschk, K. O., & Synatschk, C. (2007). *Sos!: A practical guide for leading solution-focused groups with Kids K-12.* Austin, TX: PRO-ED.

Yalom, I. D., & Leszcz, M. (2021). *The theory and practice of group psychotherapy.* New York: Basic Books.

Appendix

Glossary of Terms

Language shapes how we perceive and understand the world around us. It is constantly evolving at rapid speed. Below are important terms relevant to work with children from diverse backgrounds that are current as of writing this book. Websites such as racialequitytools.org/glossary, hrc.org/resources/glossary-of-terms, LGBTQhealth.ca and dictionary.apa.org offer up-to-date resources about identity and multiculturalism. They are tools clinicians can use to stay current, inclusive and equitable in language and practice.

Ableism   Policies and structures that reinforce the idea that to be able-bodied is the default of all humans, and to have a physical disability is unexpected or out of the norm. An example of ableism might be the assumption that all can use a set a stairs to access a voting office.

Agender   Somebody who does not identify with any gender expression or identity. May also be called gender neutral or genderless (Killermann, 2017).

Androgyny   A gender expression that has elements of both masculinity and femininity (Killermann, 2017).

Anti-Racism   A commitment to challenge and eradicate racism in all its forms by dismantling racist institutions, holding others accountable, pursuing justice, centering the voices of the oppressed, and continually re-committing the self to learning and growing.

Aromantic   Often abbreviated as 'Aro,' aromantic people have little or no romantic attraction to others. They may still have a sexual attraction to others (aromantic sexual) or find themselves uninterested in a sexual relationship (aromantic asexual).

Asexual   Often abbreviated as 'Ace,' asexual people feel little or no sexual attraction to others. This does not preclude their interest in a romantic relationship or partnership.

Bi-curious   Referring to a heterosexual person who is interested in having a romantic or sexual experience with a person of the same gender.

BIPOC   An acronym that stands for Black, Indigenous, and People of Color.

Bisexual   A person who is sexually and/or romantically attracted to other genders, as well as one's own.

Bottom Surgery   Sometimes called sex reassignment surgery, bottom surgery is for people whose reproductive organs do not fit their gender identity. A bottom surgery is a procedure meant to alter or remove sexual organs in order to fit the physical appearance and function of one's identified gender and sex.

Cisgender   A person is considered cisgender, or 'cis,' when they have the privilege of identifying comfortably within the societally sanctioned boundaries of gender expression, behavior, pronouns, and identification of their sex at birth.

Closeted   Sometimes referred to instead as being 'in the closet,' closeted people have not yet shared their gender identities and/or sexual orientations with their friends, family, work, or communities. They may be 'in the closet' due to fear of reactions, discrimination, persecution, shame, religion, etc.

Coming Out   Refers to the act of telling family, friends, work, and/or the community about one's gender identity and/or sexual orientation.

Cultural Appropriation   "Theft of cultural elements—including symbols, art, language, customs, etc.—for one's own use, commodification, or profit, often without understanding, acknowledgement, or respect for its value in the original culture. This often results from the assumption of a dominant (i.e. white) culture's right to take other cultural elements." (RacialEquityTools.org, 2022)

Cultural Bias:

1   Cultural biases occur when one has an incorrect (perhaps overly positive or overly negative) view of a particular cultural group or issue. Cultural biases have many sources, and are often a result of sociocultural messages, moral beliefs, inherited attitudes, and community beliefs (Hook, Davis, Owen, & DeBlaere, 2017).

2   Cultural biases are often unconscious, engrained attitudes and responses towards people, practices, and situations. Cultural biases in a clinician can be difficult to detect, but may be manifest through strong preferences for certain types of clientele, aversion to specific types of people or presentations, and even a vague sense of discomfort for diverse cultural presentations (Hook, Davis, Owen, & DeBlaere, 2017).

Cultural Identity   A person's cultural identity surmises their sense of belonging in terms of most salient group memberships. This might include a self-perception based on race, ethnicity, gender identity, religion, age, ability, and other broad categories of belonging.

Deadname   In the process of transitioning or otherwise embracing one's LGBTQIA+ identity, a person will often choose a name for themselves that better fits their sense of self, shedding their old name that does not fit their gender identity or self-expression. To deadname someone is to use their name assigned at birth, often in defiance of their expressed wishes or without their consent.

Demisexual   A sexual orientation that involves the necessity of an intimate emotional relationship prior to the development of sexual attraction. People who are demisexual may also identify as lesbian, gay, straight, queer, pansexual, etc.

Discrimination   Harmful behaviors and policies that target individuals based on an identity variable.

DSG   An abbreviation for Diverse Sexualities and Genders (Killermann, 2017).

Gay   A male-identifying person who is sexually and/or romantically attracted to other men.

Gender as a Construct   Gender is socially constructed, meaning it is an often-arbitrary set of rules and behaviors reinforced in a person based on their gender. For example, wearing the color pink is often considered to be for girls, despite the fact that all colors are neutral and have no objective relationship towards any gender. Gender constructs change over time and based on the geographic location of a given society.

Gender Binary   Comprised of male and female, the gender binary is a socially constructed, categorical dichotomy of gender. The gender binary describes male and female as opposites, often uses strong and rigid language to emphasize differences between genders and is reinforced by many social institutions and everyday scenarios, such as public restrooms.

Gender Dysphoria   Referring to the distress that one feels when their identified gender does not align with their biological sex, gender dysphoria is a DSM-5 diagnosis commonly given to transgender people. Though it is often a diagnosis given in the hopes of garnering gender-affirming services and resources, the diagnosis of gender dysphoria is widely considered an offensive and over-pathologizing term to describe the distress of having one's own identity under attack by social structures.

Gender Expression   Style preferences made in order to convey a sense of self in terms of gender. This may be manifest through clothing choices, hair styles, social behavior, etc., and is generally placed on the spectrum between masculine and feminine (Killermann, 2017).

Gender Fluid   A person who does not have a fixed gender identity, and fluidly shifts along the spectrum of male and female.

Gender Identity   One's internal self-identification of gender which is not outwardly visible. (American Psychological Association, 2020)

Gender Non-Conforming   A person who does not adhere to any gender script for behavior, dress, or identity.

Gender Orientation and Sexual Orientation Microaggressions   Microaggressions that subtly shame, cause discomfort, and cause feelings of unsafety for LGBTQIA+ individuals. Some common and easily identified microaggressions are flippant remarks such as, "that's so gay." More subtle and difficult to recognize due to a heteronormative culture include the assumption that every child will grow up straight, or that gender non-conforming people are just 'confused.'

Gender Queer (Non-Binary)   A person who does not identify on the gender binary, that is, as either male or female. They may consider themselves to be third gender, two-spirit, genderfluid, agender, gender -non-conforming, or something else.

GSM   An abbreviation for gender and sexual minorities (Killermann, 2017).

Heteronormativity   Often a result of cognitive bias and social conditioning, heteronormativity is the assumption that heterosexuality is the 'default' sexual orientation, and all other orientations are 'deviating' from the norm.

Heterosexism   Due to the heavily reinforced social context of heteronormativity, heterosexism describes attitudes, prejudice, and discrimination against LGBTQIA+ individuals under the assumption that they are 'deviating' from the norm of heterosexuality.

Homophobia   Prejudicial attitudes or discriminatory behavior against a person who is a member of the LGBTQIAA+ community.

Homosexuality   Describes the sexual orientation of being attracted to other members of one's sex. Due to the discrimination and prejudicial language surrounding this term, it is considered offensive to many to be called a 'homosexual.' More popular and preferred terms are lesbian or gay, though it is important to ask any individual person their preferred language.

Identities   Referring to the identity variables that we as individuals hold most salient or most important to our sense of self.

Intersectional Identity   Coined by Dr. Kimberlé Williams Crenshaw, intersectionality is the analytical framework for understanding how aspects of a person's social and political identities combine to create different modes of discrimination and privilege. (Crenshaw and Bonis, 2005).

Intersex   A person who was born with both male and female organs and anatomy, that do not fit traditional definitions of a male or female body.

Lesbian   A female-identifying person who is sexually and/or romantically attracted to other women.

LGBTQ, LGBTQIAA+   LGBTQ is an acronym for Lesbian, Gay, Bisexual, Transgender, and Queer. Becoming increasingly popular is the longer, more inclusive acronym of

LGBTQIAA+, which stands for Lesbian, Gay, Bisexual, Transgender, Intersex, Asexual, Aromantic, and other identities unlisted.

Microaggression   An insidious remark, action, attitude, or behavior that subtly communicates hostility toward a person based on their identity variables. Microaggressions are often unintentional and unnoticed by the perpetrator, but have the impact of causing discomfort, reinforcing stigma, and creating trauma for the recipient.

Neurodivergent   A term used to describe brain functioning that is different from neurotypical. This has become a preferred term in many people who have a diagnosis of ADHD or are on the autism spectrum. This term emphasizes a difference in functioning, not a deficit in functioning.

Outing   Refers to the act of disclosing someone else's gender identity or sexual orientation without their consent. This can be emotionally traumatizing for closeted individuals, as well as dangerous due to discrimination and hate.

Pansexual   A sexual orientation that involves interest for all people, without limits based on gender identities or other variables.

Polyamory   The practice of having or desiring intimate relationships with more than one partner, most often with the informed consent and assent of all involved.

Prejudice   Harmful attitudes and biases against individuals based on an identity variable.

Privilege   A special benefit or advantage only available to a particular person or group. For example, white privilege might be the ease at which a white person is granted a home loan, can access social services, or can trust that law enforcement agents will not harm them because of their skin tone.

Pronouns   A pronoun is a word that takes place of a noun, such as he/him/his, she/her/hers, and they/them. People who do not identify on the gender binary may prefer to use gender-neutral pronouns such as they/them, or ze/zir. Some people feel most comfortable in creating their own pronouns. In respecting people's gender identities and expressions, it is important to ask which pronouns they prefer and strive to use them in all interactions.

Queer   A word used to describe a large spectrum of sexual orientations and gender identities. Some people prefer the term 'queer' over 'gay.' It is important to ask for preferences, and not make assumptions.

Racism   "A form of prejudice that assumes that the members of racial categories have distinctive characteristics and that these differences result in some racial groups being inferior to others. Racism generally includes negative emotional reactions to members of the group, acceptance of negative stereotypes, and racial discrimination against individuals." (American Psychological Association, 2020).

Sapiosexual   A sexual orientation that involves attraction to one's intelligence.

Sexism   Prejudicial attitudes or discriminatory behavior against a person who identifies as female.

Sexual Orientation   Sexual orientation refers to one's attraction to others based on their preferences. Sexual orientation encapsulates lesbian, gay, bisexual, asexual, romantic, aromantic, etc. It is entirely separate from gender identity, which refers to one's sense of self in terms of gender.

Singlism   Prejudicial attitudes or discriminatory behavior against a person who is single, rather than partnered. Singlism is most negatively impactful toward people who identify as women.

Skoliosexual   A sexual orientation that involves attraction to non-binary and transgender people.

Stereotypes:

1   Stereotypes are a type of cultural bias that reduce individuals to an over-simplistic, over-generalized, or rigid understanding of who they are based on a constructed social category (Hook, Davis, Owen, & DeBlaere, 2017).

2   Stereotypes simplify perceptions and judgments. They are often exaggerated, negative rather than positive, and resistant to revision even when perceivers encounter individuals who do not fit their stereotype (American Psychological Association, 2020).

Systemic Racism   Racism that is embedded in the structure of a society, and is perpetuated by laws, policies, law enforcement, etc., that unfairly target or discriminate against a certain demographic.

Third Gender   A person who does not identify as either male or female but falls into a third category for gender.

Top Surgery   Sometimes called gender- affirming surgery, top surgery is for people whose anatomy of the torso does not fit their gender identity. A top surgery is a procedure meant to either remove breast tissue or place prosthetic breast implants.

Transgender (Trans)   A gender identity that differs from the sex assigned at birth.

Transitioning   A transgender person who is in the process of transitioning to their identified gender orientation. This might include the use of hormone replacement therapy, surgical procedures, and changing of the outward appearance in order to better express one's inward identity.

Transphobia   Prejudicial attitudes or discriminatory behavior against a person who is transgender or transitioning.

Two-Spirit   Originating in Native American, First Nation, and Indigenous cultures, a two-spirit person is one who identifies as having both a masculine and feminine spirit. Two-spirit is an umbrella term used to describe a vast number of orientations and gender identities, such as gender queer, gender fluid, gender non-conforming, etc. members of the Indigenous community.

White Fragility   "A state in which even a minimum amount of racial stress becomes intolerable [for white people], triggering a range of defensive moves. These moves include the outward display of emotions such as anger, fear, and guilt, and behaviors such as argumentation, silence, and leaving the stress-inducing situation. These behaviors, in turn, function to reinstate white racial equilibrium." (DiAngelo, 2011, p. 1).

White Silence   In racial dialogue, white individuals keeping perspectives hidden and therefor unable to be explored, discussed, or challenged while providing a sense of psychological safety.

Index

Note: **Bold** page numbers refer to tables and *italic* page numbers refer to figures.

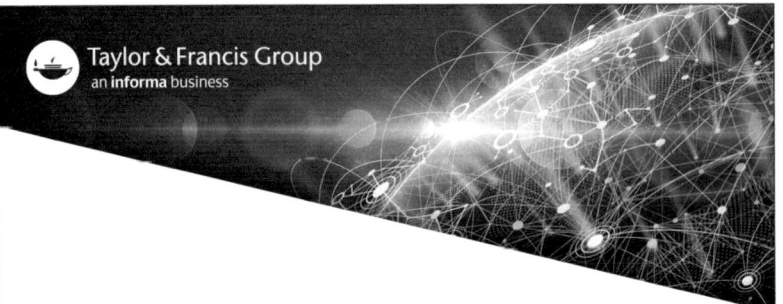
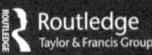
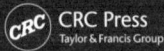